Veterinary Anatomy and Physiology

Edited by Catrin Sian Rutland and Valentina Kubale

Published in London, United Kingdom

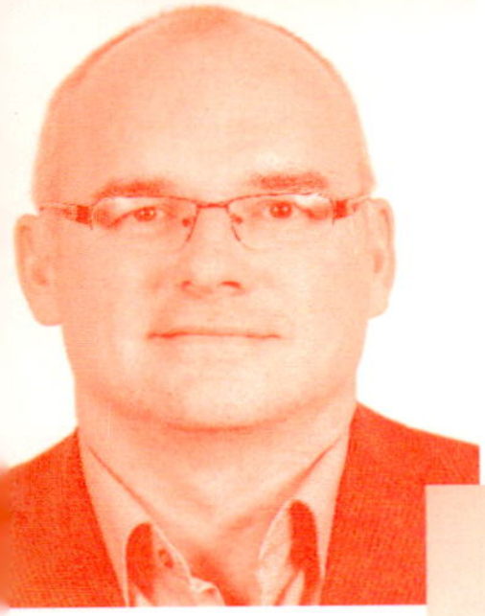

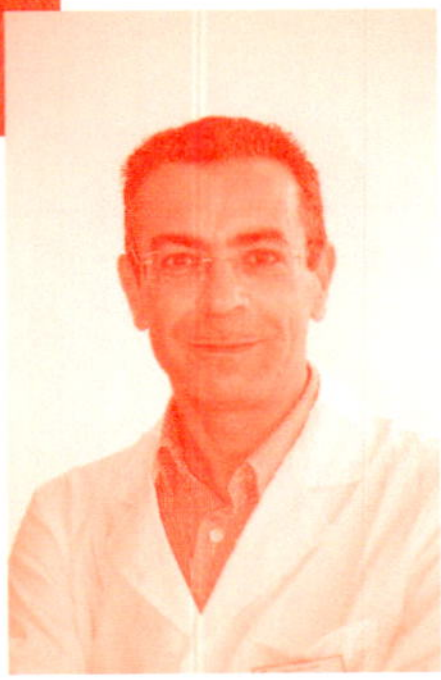

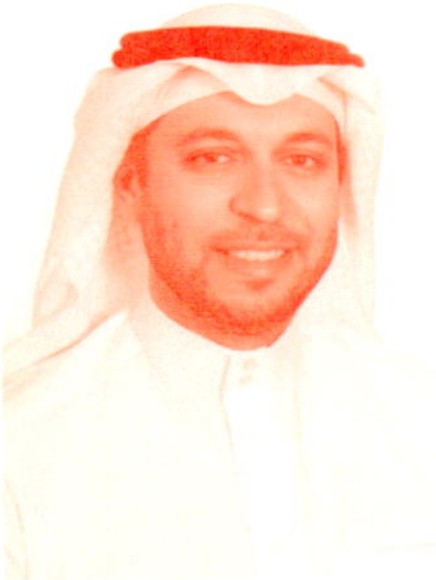

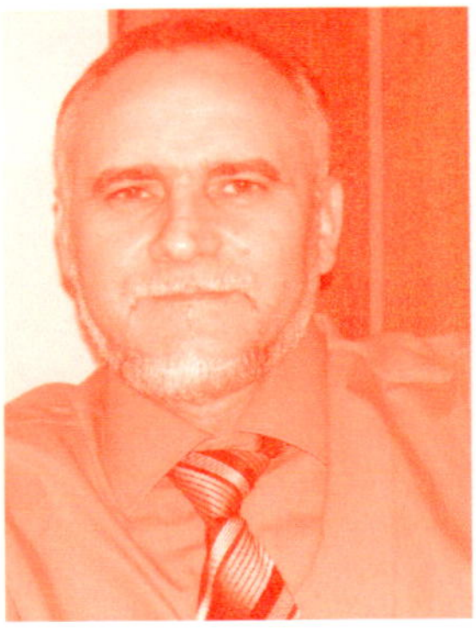

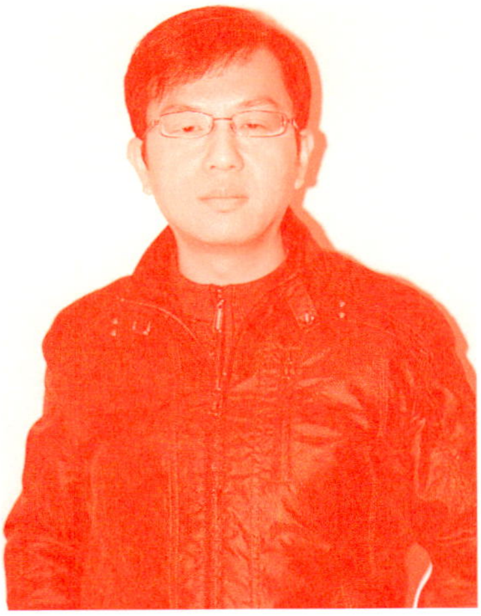

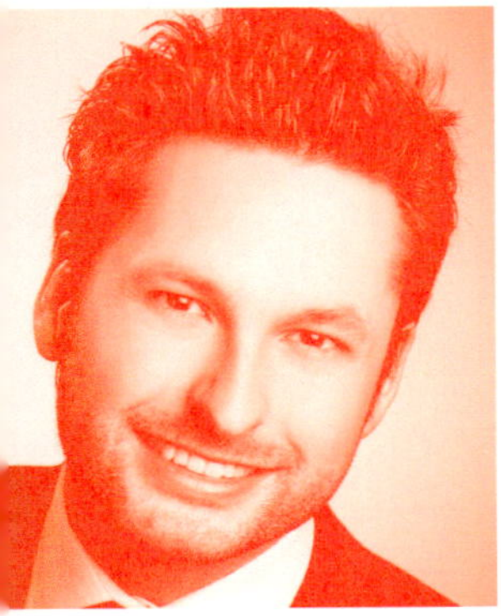

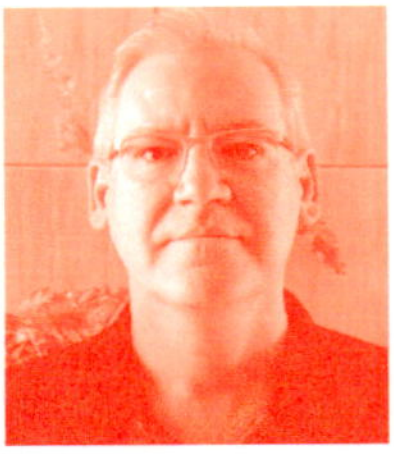

IntechOpen

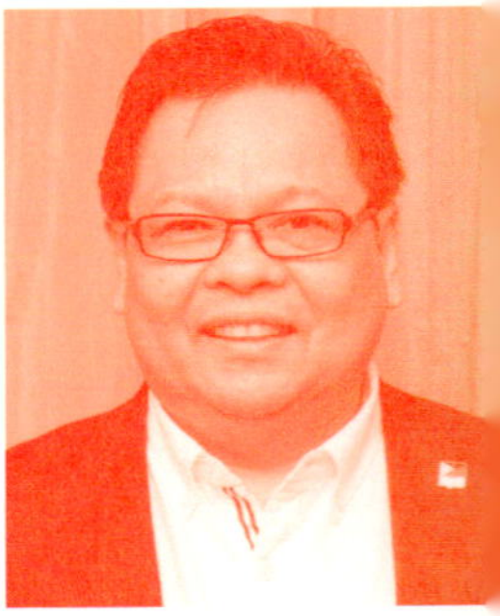

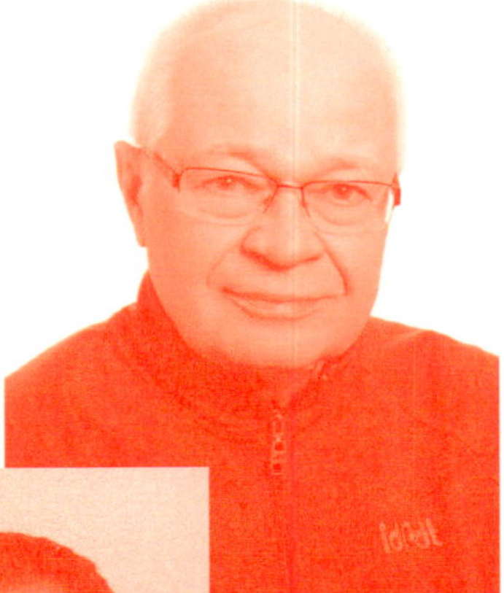

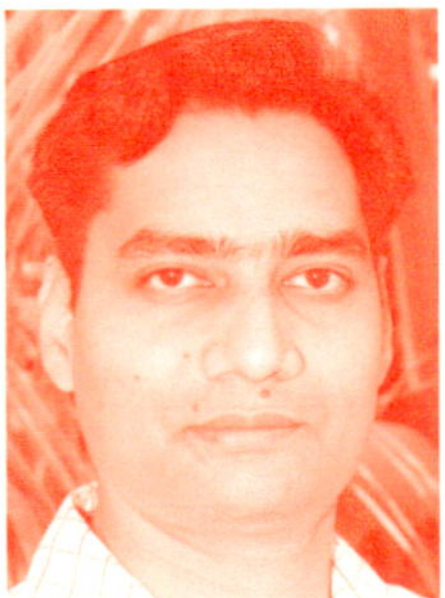

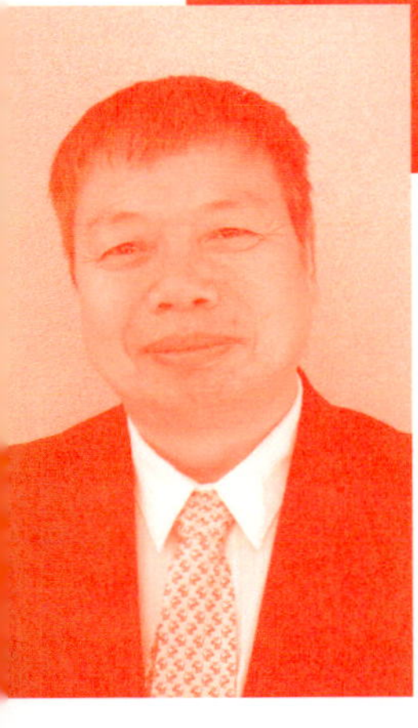

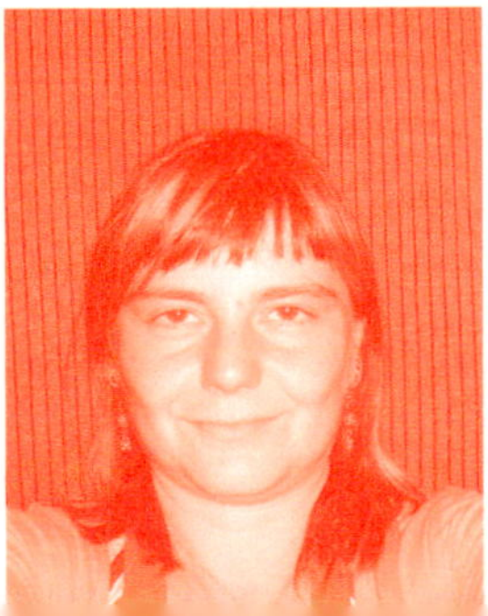

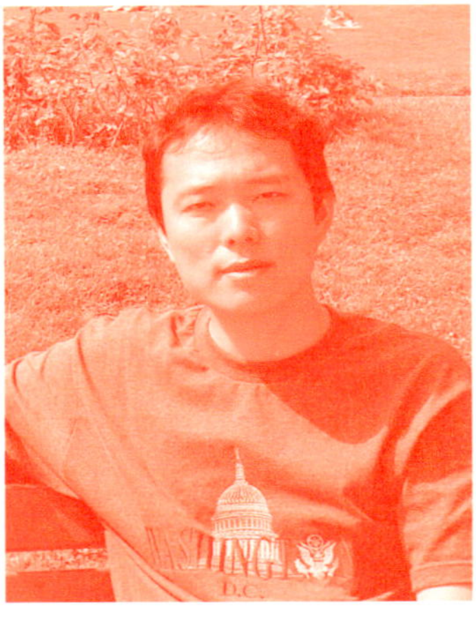

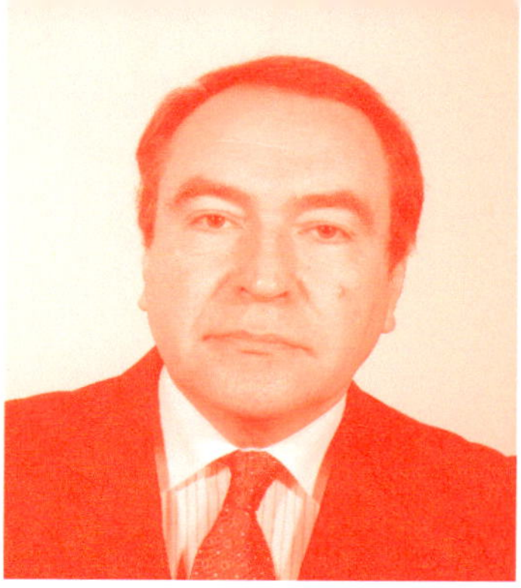
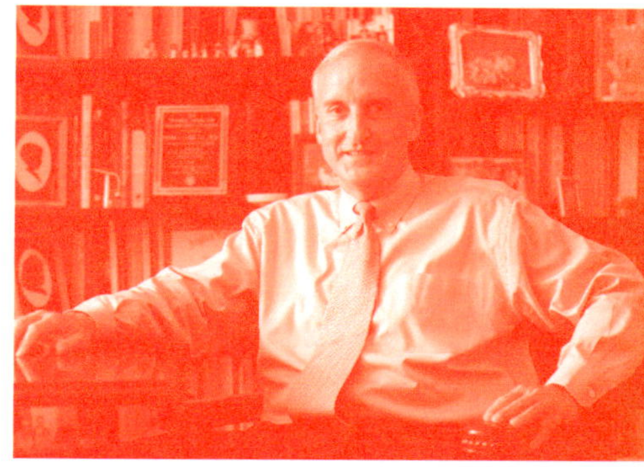
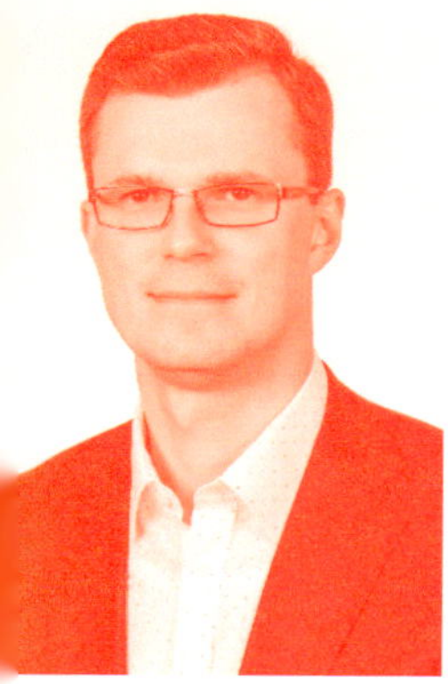
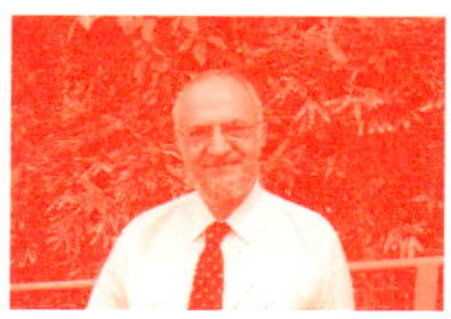
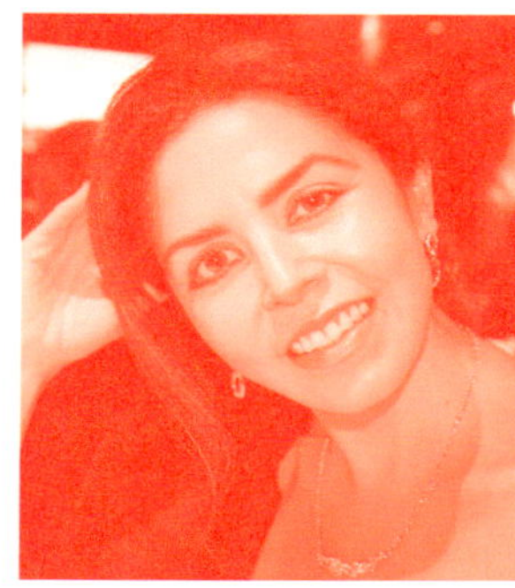

Supporting open minds since 2005

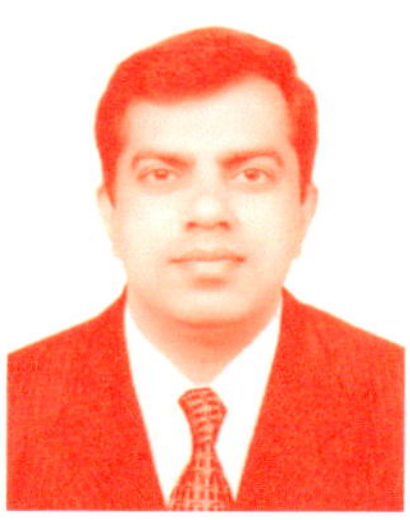
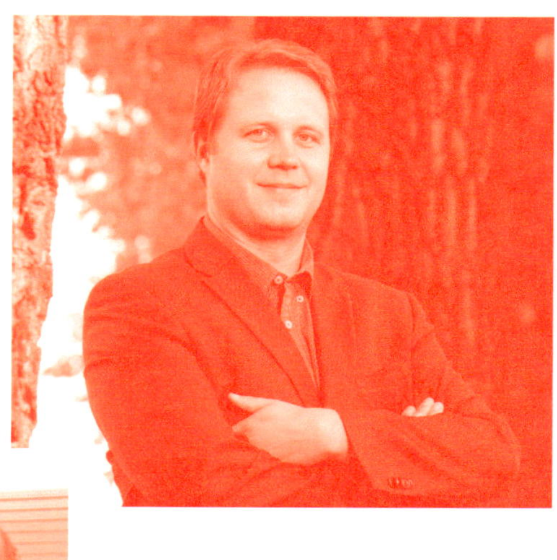
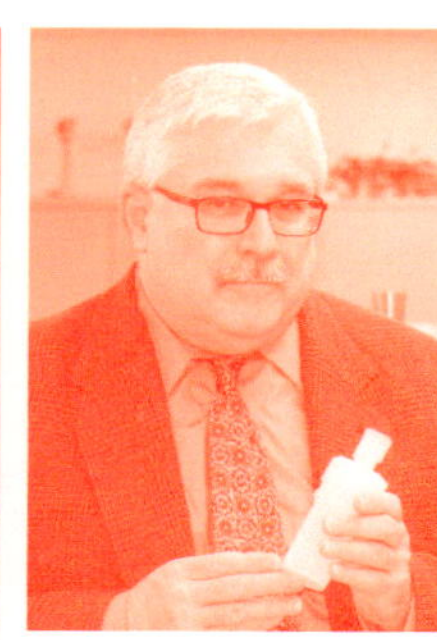
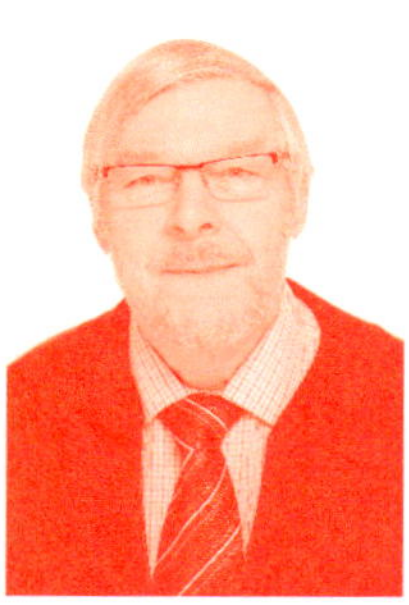
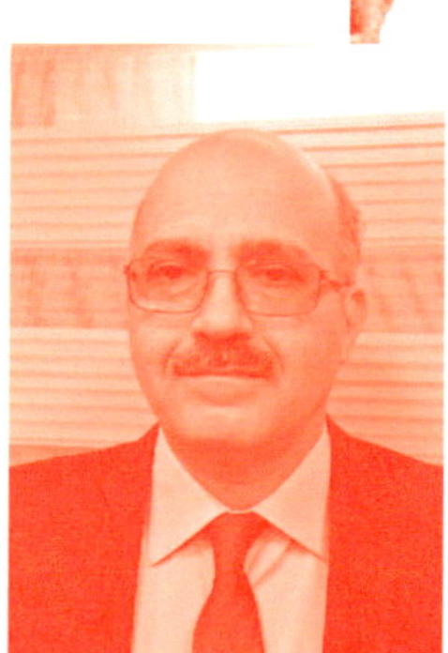
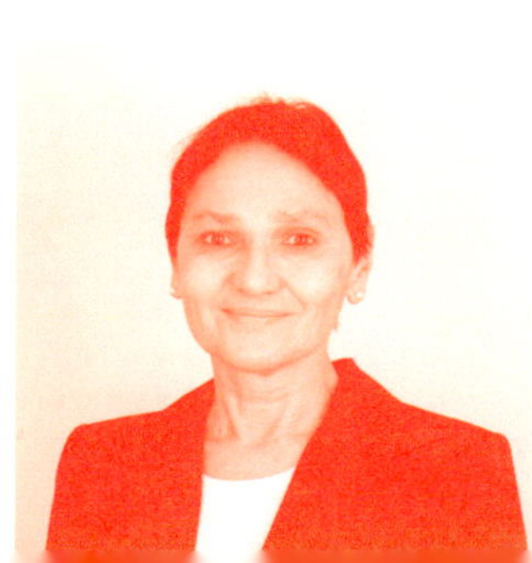
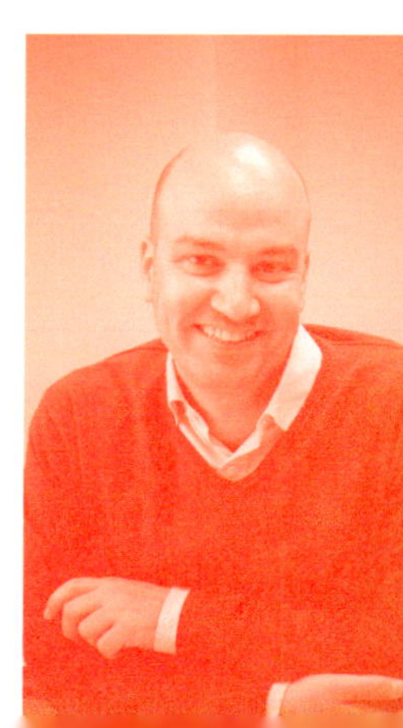

Veterinary Anatomy and Physiology
http://dx.doi.org/10.5772/intechopen.73942
Edited by Catrin Sian Rutland and Valentina Kubale

Part of IntechOpen Book Series: Veterinary Medicine and Science, Volume 2
Book Series Editor: Rita Payan-Carreira

Contributors
Dmitrii Oleinikov, Carlos Eduardo Fonseca-Alves, Antonio Fernando Leis Filho, Ramzi Al-Agele, Catrin Sian Rutland, Emily Paul, Valentina Kubale Dvojmoč, Cyril Rauch, Craig Sturrock, Samir El-Gendy, Emma Cousins, Clara Bailey, James Nguhiu-Mwangi, Peter Mbithi, Meskerem Adamu, Maria De Lurdes Pinto, Diana Fernandes

First published in London, United Kingdom, 2019 by IntechOpen
IntechOpen is the global imprint of INTECHOPEN LIMITED, registered in England and Wales, registration number: 11086078, The Shard, 25th floor, 32 London Bridge Street
London, SE19SG – United Kingdom
Printed in Croatia

British Library Cataloguing-in-Publication Data
A catalogue record for this book is available from the British Library

Additional hard copies can be obtained from orders@intechopen.com

Veterinary Anatomy and Physiology
Edited by Catrin Sian Rutland and Valentina Kubale
p. cm.
Print ISBN 978-1-78985-705-4
Online ISBN 978-1-78985-706-1
ISSN 2632-0517

For EU product safety concerns:
IN TECH d.o.o., Prolaz Marije Krucifikse Kozulić 3, 51000 Rijeka, Croatia, info@intechopen.com or visit our website at intechopen.com.

IntechOpen Book Series

Veterinary Medicine and Science

Volume 2

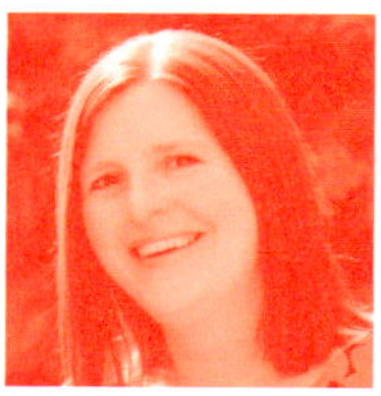

Catrin Rutland is an Associate Professor of Anatomy and Developmental Genetics at the University of Nottingham, UK. Catrin completed her Degree, Masters then PhD (University of Derby, Technische Universität München, and University of Nottingham), and undertook a postdoctoral research fellowship at the School of Medicine before accepting a tenure in Veterinary Medicine and Science. She also achieved her MMedSci (Medical Education) and PGCHE. Catrin is the author of over 100 research papers/books/abstracts. She is a board member of the European Association of Veterinary Anatomists, Fellow of the Anatomical Society and Galton Institute, Senior Fellow of the Higher Education Academy, and member of the British Society for Developmental Biology, Society for Reproduction and Fertility, and Society of Cancer Epigenetics. Orcid: https://orcid.org/0000-0002-2009-4898. Website https://www.nottingham.ac.uk/vet/people/catrin.rutland

Editor of Volume 2:
Catrin Rutland
University of Nottingham, UK

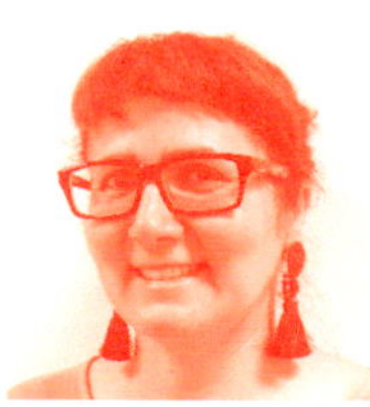

Valentina Kubale is Assistant Professor of Veterinary Medicine at the Veterinary Faculty, University of Ljubljana, Slovenia. Since graduating from the Veterinary faculty, she obtained her PhD in 2007, and collaborated with the Department of Pharmacology, University of Copenhagen, Denmark. She continued as a postdoctoral fellow at the University of Copenhagen with a Lundbeck Foundation fellowship. She is the editor of two books and author/coauthor of 21 articles in peer-reviewed scientific journals, 13 book chapters, and 54 communications at scientific congresses. Since 2008 she has been the Editor Assistant for the Slovenian Veterinary Research journal. She is a member of the Slovenian Biochemical Society, the Endocrine Society, the European Association of Veterinary Anatomists, and the Society for Laboratory Animals, where she is a board member.

Editor of Volume 2:
Valentina Kubale
University of Ljubljana, Slovenia

Book Series Editor:
Rita Payan-Carreira
University of Évora, Portugal

Scope of the Series

Paralleling similar advances in the medical field, astounding advances occurred in the Veterinary Medicine and Science in recent decades, fostering a better support to animal health and more humane animal production, a better understanding of the physiology of endangered species, to improve the assisted reproductive technologies or the pathogenesis of certain diseases, where animals can be used as models for human diseases (like cancer, degenerative diseases or fertility), and even as a guarantee of public health. Bridging the Human, Animal and Environmental health, the holistic and integrative "One Health" concept intimately associates the developments within those fields, projecting its advancements into practice.

This book series aims to tackle a variety of fields in the animal-related medicine and sciences, providing thematic volumes, high quality and significance in the field, directed to researchers and postgraduates. It aims to give us a glimpse into the new accomplishments in the Veterinary Medicine and Science field. By addressing hot topics in veterinary sciences, we aim to gather authoritative texts within each issue of this series, providing in-depth overviews and analysis for graduates, academics and practitioners and foreseeing a deeper understanding of the subject. Forthcoming texts, written and edited by experienced researchers from both industry and academia, will also discuss scientific challenges faced today in Veterinary Medicine and Science. In brief, we hope that books in this series will provide accessible references for those interested or working in this field and encourage learning in a range of different topics.

Contents

Preface

Understanding veterinary anatomy and physiology is an essential part of animal medicine and welfare. This book contains both literature reviews and recent research into topics ranging from cardiovascular medicine through to conservation of species such as the horse, dog, cow, chicken, and reptiles. As editors we are both practicing anatomy and physiology researchers and teachers and therefore we have strived to ensure that every chapter is accessible to everyone. Whether you are a veterinary professional, student, researcher, animal owner, or simply have an interest in veterinary anatomy and physiology, we hope you will find a number of interesting chapters in this book.

The chapter "Introduction to Veterinary Anatomy and Physiology" covers a brief history and background of veterinary anatomy and physiology from the past up until the present day. This book is part of IntechOpen's *Women in Science Book Collection*; therefore, there is also an introduction on the roles and present standing of women in veterinary medicine, anatomy, and physiology. The next section covers the hoof and musculoskeletal system and contains chapters on "The Anatomy, Histology and Physiology of the Healthy and Lame Equine Hoof" and "Macroscopic, Radiographic and Histopathologic Changes of Claws with Laminitis-related Disorders in Zero-Grazed Dairy Cows." Both chapters highlight the latest research and techniques used to further understand the hoof and disorders affecting horses and cows, which are of vital importance to animal health.

In the cardiorespiratory and reproductive systems section, three chapters cover "Myocardial Metabolism," "Anatomy, Histology and Physiology of the Canine Prostate Gland," and "Health Limitations and Ethno-veterinary Practices of Small Scale and Backyard Chicken Production in Some Selected Regions of Ethiopia." Much is published about intensive farming and large-scale production, but understanding smaller farming techniques and practices is vital in a world where many rely on this as a food source.

The final section covers exotics, wildlife, and conservation. Two chapters explore "Veterinarian's Role in Conservation Medicine and Animal Welfare," an increasingly important area of research in our changing world, and "Reptilian Skin and Its Special Histological Structures," an area that has fewer publications but is important not only in understanding wildlife but also because the popularity of reptiles as companion animals has increased dramatically over the decades.

The chapter contributors are experts in their field from across the world and have used a number of graphics throughout to illustrate their work. The latest microcomputed tomography, histological techniques, X-rays, photographs, and schematics are used to help describe the features discussed.

Dr. Catrin Sian Rutland
University of Nottingham, UK

Dr. Valentina Kubale
University of Ljubljana, Slovenia

Section 1

Introduction to Veterinary Anatomy and Physiology

Chapter 1

Introductory Chapter: Veterinary Anatomy and Physiology

Valentina Kubale, Emma Cousins, Clara Bailey, Samir A.A. El-Gendy and Catrin Sian Rutland

1. History of veterinary anatomy and physiology

The anatomy of animals has long fascinated people, with mural paintings depicting the superficial anatomy of animals dating back to the Palaeolithic era [1]. However, evidence suggests that the earliest appearance of scientific anatomical study may have been in ancient Babylonia, although the tablets upon which this was recorded have perished and the remains indicate that Babylonian knowledge was in fact relatively limited [2].

As such, with early exploration of anatomy documented in the writing of various papyri, ancient Egyptian civilisation is believed to be the origin of the anatomist [3]. With content dating back to 3000 BCE, the Edwin Smith papyrus demonstrates a recognition of cerebrospinal fluid, meninges and surface anatomy of the brain, whilst the Ebers papyrus describes systemic function of the body including the heart and vasculature, gynaecology and tumours [4]. The Ebers papyrus dates back to around 1500 BCE; however, it is also thought to be based upon earlier texts. In the early third century, a school of anatomy was founded in Alexandria and became the first of its kind carrying out human dissection [5]. It was based on the Greek system, following Hippocratic teachings. Hippocrates (ca. 460–370 BCE) had described the human brain as being in two halves divided by a thin vertical membrane, as it was in other animals. The most renowned Alexandrian physicians were Herophilus and Erasistratus. Many graduates of this medical school travelled and practiced throughout the Mediterranean basin.

Many renowned Greek anatomists studied in Alexandria, but as Egypt entered a slow decline, developments in Greek philosophical and scientific culture began to surpass all current knowledge of anatomy and physiology [4]. The early scientist Alcmaeon of Croton, a Greek medic is widely credited for attributing the mind to the brain in around 500 BCE [6]. He also observed that the arteries and veins in his animal dissections appeared dissimilar to each other [7]. Herophilus progressed these theories around the brain and identified the organ as the centre of the nervous system [8]. Herophilus was born in 335 BCE, studied in Alexandria and remained there during the reigns of the first two Ptolemaios Pharaohs and is said to be the first anatomist to perform a systematic dissection of the human body. Erasistratus concentrated on physiology and mechanisms rather than the pure anatomy. This was not always a popular method of describing the body during either his life or later on.

Roman Marcus Aurelius (161–180 CE) highlighted that physicians were more likely to maim or kill their patients they were not aware of the anatomy required. He was famous for his mission to understand anatomy and physiology in a range of animals extending from monkeys and snakes to cattle and cats, in both adults and young. He even noted the similarities between macaques and humans. Ultimately it was the Greek Aristotle who became known as the father of comparative anatomy through his dissections performed on a variety of animals, including mammals, reptiles and insects [9].

Moving into the second century, the Greek anatomist Galen pioneered a number of anatomical and physiological theories, mainly through animal dissection [5]. Galen was responsible for the discovery of the recurrent laryngeal nerve [10], and had many advanced theories on wound healing [11]. His work remained influential in anatomical and physiological science for fifteen centuries and allowed significant advancements in medicine [12].

In the following years, until the twelfth century, much of the anatomical study that took place was therapeutically focussed and completed following the written works of early authors such as Galen [13]. The appearance of anatomist Mondino dei Luzzi in the thirteenth century induced progression in anatomical and physiological study based upon his work with human cadaver dissection [14]. Whilst Andreas Vesalius, an important figure in the Renaissance, pushed forward physiological study with accurate accounts of the mechanics of pulmonary ventilation, among many other revelations in his 1543 work entitled 'De Humani Corporis Fabrica' [15].

A number of years later, born in 1578 in England, William Harvey was the first to correctly describe the circulatory system, identifying the blood flow returning to the heart and the heart acting as a muscular pump [16]. Harvey also proposed the idea of capillary anastomoses joining the arterial and venous systems, although their existence was not proven until after his death by Marcello Malpighi in 1661 [16].

The eighteenth and nineteenth centuries saw dissection became a more prominent feature in anatomical study, when William Hunter encouraged students to carry out their own dissection on cadavers. This however led to 'body-snatching', and as a result, The Anatomy Act (1832) was enforced in order to regulate the acquisition of human cadaveric material [17]. This regulation favoured the anatomy schools based in hospitals and as such, the professionalisation of the science was observed [18].

At the present time, anatomy and physiology are unarguably fundamental aspects of medical education and can be taught in many ways including dissection, 'self-directed learning' and 'problem based learning' [19]. Recent developments in technology have allowed digital anatomical models to be implemented into university curricula, allowing wider access to the study of anatomy for the contemporary student [20].

2. Imaging technology within anatomy and physiology

In the days of the first anatomists and physiologists discussed above, fewer tools and techniques were available to allow visualisation of the body. Over the years many techniques have been developed by scientists that have been essential for veterinary and human anatomists and physiologists alike. Dissection and drawing were always essential skills and are still used today. As the first microscopes were developed the ability to see within the tissue and cell both anatomy and physiology were advanced, alongside medical practice. The first modern microscope developed by Hans and Zacharias Janssen in 1590 has certainly changed over the years [21]. There is also much evidence to suggest the use and theories on early microscopes and lens magnification from early China 4000 years ago and even the ancient Greeks and Romans. Hooke also designed a microscope and wrote the now famous 'Micrographia' and Antonie van Leeuwenhoek-the Father of the Microscope developed this work and his publications to the Royal Society were validated by non-other than Hooke [21]. The modern microscope has advanced greatly with optical microscopy utilising a nonlinear optical phenomenon, electron microscopy, confocal microscopy and even hand held microscopes now available for the pursuit of anatomical, physiological and medical research and diagnosis.

Since the discovery of X-rays, developments in medical imaging have provided a powerful tool of investigation allowing visualisation of the body in detail never before seen [22]. The combination of postmortem cadaveric dissection and imaging techniques of live patients has proven to be an important technique in understanding the anatomy and physiology of the live animal [23].

1895 saw X-rays observed for the first time by German physicist Wilhelm Roentgen [24]. By imaging his wife's hand, Roentgen deducted that bone and metal were opaque on radiographs and medical uses of the technology quickly followed [25]. Marie Curie used a portable X-ray unit to visualise skeletal trauma in soldiers on French battlefields [22]. Whilst, the use of X-ray crystallography was vital in understanding the genetic code, which in turn has had an enormous impact upon the understanding of physiology [24].

In later years, Godfrey Hounsfield expanded the use of X-rays by developing computer software that could integrate multiple radiographic images to give a three-dimensional view inside the body [26]. This was the discovery of computed tomography (CT) [27]. CT had a significant advantage over radiographs alone as it allowed the distinction of different soft tissue types to be visualised [28]. In 1971 the first CT scan of patient took place, successfully scanning the brain for a tumour in the frontal lobe [29]. The invention of CT had vital practical applications, and as a result, Hounsfield was awarded the Nobel Prize for Physiology or Medicine in 1979 [26].

The risks of using ionising radiation were acknowledged, particularly regarding imaging of the foetus, and as such, a reduction in use of X-rays was seen and replacement with ultrasonography and magnetic resonance imaging occurred [24]. Ian Donald pioneered the use of ultrasound in obstetrics and gynaecology in a paper published in 1958 [30]. Since this time, two-dimension ultrasound techniques have been significantly developed and three-dimension ultrasound can map and quantify blood flow [31]. Ultrasound has been a critical milestone for medical imaging and a fundamental method of non-invasive research [32].

However, the breakthrough of magnetic resonance imaging (MRI) has become a vital diagnostic and research tool in recent years [33]. Nuclear magnetic resonance was originally discovered by Felix Bloch and Edward Purcell in 1946 and formed a foundation for the development of modern day MRI. The use of NMR was developed by Paul Lauterbur when he applied gradients to magnetic fields to create a two-dimensional image and Sir Peter Mansfield developed methods of/slice selection and creating and interpreting images. These advance resulted in the development of MRI as we know it now [33] and the men shared the Nobel Prize in Medicine or Physiology in 2003. MRI is an important medical imaging tool, using no ionising radiation and providing a practical alternative to invasive procedures [34].

A recent development in imaging is that of imaging mass spectrometry that allows tissue samples to be visualised on a molecular level without labelling with chemicals or antibodies [35]. The mass spectrometry imaging technology was developed by a group of physicists, including Caprioli and the technique is particularly sensitive for use on proteins and peptides [36]. This technology however cannot map the transcriptome and a new technique, mass spectrometric imaging, has been developed as a result [37].

Moving forwards, it is predicted that radiography will progress to tomography based methods as opposed to projection based and molecular imaging may become more popular [38, 39]. It is also very likely that the field of imaging will continue to develop and give us deeper insights into anatomy and physiology [38]. Imaging is a key part of both anatomy and physiology but by no means the only tool used. We can see the advances made in imaging but many tools have either developed over the years or been discovered in more recent years. Genetics has revolutionised the worlds of anatomy and physiology for example. Understanding cellular and molecular biology alongside anatomy and physiology has become essential in the research we undertake today. Anatomy seeks to understand the structure, location and composition of the parts within organisms and their relationships with each other. Physiology seeks to understand the functions and processes of organisms, how they work and ultimately assist with understanding and treating diseases and disorders. Therefore whilst imaging is essential for both of these practices, the continued development and discovery of more tools are needed in order to further our research. Much of the work in this book uses these techniques, or a combination of them in the pursuit of advancing anatomical and physiological knowledge and understanding.

3. Women in veterinary medicine, anatomy and physiology

This book is part of the IntechOpen's 'Women in Sciences Book Collection'; therefore, it seems appropriate to discuss some of the women who have worked in anatomy and physiology, the history of women in veterinary medicine and the present day situation. As with most of the sciences, the majority of people already discussed in this introductory chapter are men. It is not that women were not making advances in science, rather that they were historically less likely to be working in these areas.

Claude Bourgelat founded the first veterinary school in Lyon 1762 [40]. The UK's first veterinary school, The Veterinary College in London, was not opened until 1791 [41]. At that time, there were no regulations to study veterinary medicine and practitioners often had no formal training [42, 43]. Fifty years later the Royal Charter 1844 allowed the Royal College of Veterinary Surgeons to be created, giving the profession recognition [44, 45]. The Veterinary Surgeons Act 1881 distinguished qualified practitioners from those who were unqualified [45]. Veterinary work was originally centred around the horse, with many veterinarians employed in the army and public services [41, 46]. When engines evolved and horses less in demand, the number of equine veterinarians diminished so the profession then began to focus on farm animals and livestock [41, 46, 47]. During the mid-twentieth century the interest in companion animal care increased and the small animal sector grew [46].

The number of women in anatomy and physiology research has grown over the years. These women have a background either in veterinary medicine or in the basic sciences (biology, anatomy, animal science) or even transfer from human medicine and anatomy to veterinary research. The first UK female veterinary surgeon was Aleen Cust who completed her training in 1900 at Edinburgh Veterinary College. At this time, the Royal College of Veterinary Surgeons refused her membership and therefore Cust could not obtain a diploma from the RCVS [48]. It was not until 1922 when Cust obtained her full RCVS membership aided by The Sex Disqualification (Removal) Act of 1919, which forbade the discrimination of women [48].

Mary Brancker was the first woman president of the British Veterinary Association and a key founding member in the Society of Women Veterinary Surgeons [49, 50]. Brancker was incredibly influential and she obtained an OBE for her work during the foot and mouth disease outbreak in 1967–1968. Additionally she was awarded CBE for her contribution to animal health and welfare in 2000 [49. The influence of women in veterinary medicine continued to grow as Dame Olga Uvarov became the first woman president of the RCVS in 1976 [51].

In recent years, the veterinary profession has seen a substantial increase in the number of female veterinary surgeons, despite being a previously male-dominated occupation. Removal of gender discrimination, such as the Women's Education Act of 1974 in the UK and similar movements and laws around the world, has been fundamental in allowing females to gain admission to veterinary colleges [52, 53]. In 2006, 51% of UK working veterinary surgeons were female [54] and by 2014, this number had increased to 57.6% [55]. Women now represent around 80% of veterinary medicine and science graduates in many countries including the United Kingdom, Slovenia and the United States of America however there is still thought to be a divide in the types of areas they later decide to work in [52]. The decrease in the number of men applying to veterinary colleges is thought to be due to declining salaries and pre-emptive flight—men are discouraged from entering the profession due to the increasing number of women [56, 57]. Although there are many historical reasons why fewer women entered the profession, it is clear that throughout the world the numbers of women entering the profession are increasing.

The demographic shift of the profession is not unique to the UK—it has occurred globally. In 1963 there were as few as 277 qualified female veterinary surgeons in the United States [58]. In 2017 females accounted for 55.7% of the total United States veterinary professionals [59]. Similarly, statistics in Canada showed that, in 2017, 55.8% of veterinary surgeons were women [60] and females now make up 80% of the Canadian veterinary student population [61]. In Australia 2010, 50% of registered veterinarians were female [44].

In other countries, feminisation of the veterinary profession has occurred at a slower rate. In Turkey, the proportion of female graduates was 26.2% between 2000 and 2005 compared to only 4.9% between 1975 and 1979 [62]. In Iran, women were previously banned from studying veterinary medicine. However since these restrictions were lifted the number of female veterinary students increased to 51.1% in 2003 [63].

In the past, many veterinary colleges stated they did not want female admissions—many believed women were not strong enough to handle large animals and were too sentimental to cope with the challenges of the work [43, 53]. Today sentimentality is considered vital in veterinary medicine, particularly when working with emotional clientele in companion animal practice [43]. The trend that more female than male graduates enter companion animal practice [43, 59, 60, 64] has posed the question whether the large animal industry will suffer [57]. However it has been highlighted the use of safer chemical restraints has eliminated the significance of physical strength, making the large animal sector more appealing to woman practitioners [53].

Despite increased numbers of female veterinary surgeons, practice ownership is still largely male dominated [46, 54, 65]. Only 6.5% of UK female veterinary surgeons held a director position in 2014 [66]. It is widely known that employees earn lower incomes in comparison to practice owners and directors [46, 65, 67]. The under-representation of women in practice ownership and increasingly low incomes of female employees could potentially stagnate the income of the entire profession [43, 46, 56, 57, 68]. Although, one study found that 73% of UK female veterinary students aspired to own a practice after graduating [69], indicating that women do wish to take on senior roles in a veterinary business; however may not get the opportunity. Therefore there is a significant wage gap between male and female veterinary surgeons but this also extends to starting wages. Full time starting salaries of male veterinarians were $56,433 compared to the female veterinarian mean full time starting salary of $48,722 in the United States [64]. One of our recent reviews also looked at women in academia in the sciences, including veterinary medicine and the basic sciences in order to show details such as reduced career progression, reduced income and other gender inequalities still present in academic institutions throughout the world [70].

At the beginning of this introductory chapter we listed just a few of the anatomists and physiologists from throughout history but documenting women in anatomy and physiology is sometimes more difficult. For many years women were not expected, allowed or encouraged to undertake education or the sciences in general. A quick look at Wikipedia (as of November 2018) showed just 10 pages for 'women anatomists' and 29 for 'women physiologists' [71]. It is difficult to correlate with the pages for men as these are not a subcategory in their own rights. Some of the anatomists and physiologists included on this site are international renowned, whilst others have made huge advances but are less well known. Italian Alessandra Giliani (1307–1326) was the first documented female anatomist although there is some debate around this matter, but she not only created prosections but was also a surgical assistant and is said to have undertaken research into the circulatory system [72]. In many ways the Italian universities really started a more modern revolution in that women were allowed to study and become academics. Anna Morandi Manzolini (1714–1774) worked as a professor at the University of Bologna as an anatomist, became a member of the Russian Royal Scientific Association and the British Royal Society [73]. Many years later Marion Bidder (1862–1932) an English physiologist became the first woman to do independent research at Cambridge University and also the first women to present her own work at the Royal Society [74]. Vera Mikhaĭlovna Danchakof (1879–1950) a Russian anatomist worked in the field and is often known as 'the mother of stem cells' [75]. At a similar time Katharine Julia Scott Bishop (1889–1975) born in the United States of America co-discovered vitamin E [76]. Around this time more women were able to work within universities worldwide. Ruth Bowden (1915–2001) from India became known for her work on striated muscle disease and leprosy [77] and Ruth Smith Lloyd (1917–1995) was the first African- American to achieve a PhD in anatomy working on fertility in both anatomical and physiological terms. Marian Diamond (1926–2017) born in the United States of America is often considered as one of the founders of modern neuroscience [78]. Mary Anne Frey (1945-present) was not only the chief scientist at NASA but also made real advances in the effects of gravity on the body [79]. Although it is not usual to source from Wikipedia, the aforementioned links may be useful for people interested in obtaining further information about these scientists.

Naturally over the last century a number of women have also won Nobel Prizes. These include Gerty Theresa Cori, Rosalyn Yalow, Barbara McClintock, Rita Levi-Montalcini, Gertrude B. Elion, Christiane Nüsslein-Volhard, Linda B. Buck, Françoise Barré-Sinoussi, Carol W. Greider, Elizabeth H. Blackburn, May-Britt Moser, and Youyou Tu [80]. Whilst not all of these scientists were specifically veterinary anatomists or physiologists, many did use these disciplines to help with their discoveries ranging from therapies against malaria, discovery of HIV, understanding chromosomes and DNA, understanding the olfactory system, early embryonic development, drug treatment discoveries, growth factors and countless other essential works throughout their lives.

The world is not filled with Nobel Prize winning scientists or pages on Wikipedia. It is difficult to ascertain the exact numbers of women in anatomy and physiology worldwide as this encompass both veterinary surgeons and scientists from the biological and biomedical fields. Many teach undergraduate and post graduate students, undertake research, work in industry and have other roles in educational establishments. International organisations such as the World, European, African and American Associations of Veterinary Anatomists and the international nomenclature committees all have female members, committee members and/or presidents and certainly other leading societies have similar situations [81–84]. Looking at the International Union of Physiological Sciences, Federation of

European Physiological Societies, American Physiology Society, Federation of the Asian and Oceanian Physiological Societies and the societies that they represent a similar pattern is observed [85–89].

Attending conferences, looking at the committee members, fellows, members, organising and scientific committees and looking at the literature being produced through books and peer reviewed papers it is clear that women now take substantial leading roles in the instruction of, and research into, veterinary physiology and anatomy. It has to be noted that many societies now also have equality officers (or equivalent) and even sub committees concentrating on women in science, for example the American Physiological Society has a 'Women in Physiology' committee to promote excellence in mentoring, to promote the visibility and success of women in physiology among many other aims [87]. Whilst specific committees, networks or similar activities are not always evident it is important to note that over the centuries and more recent decades the people involved in the sciences in general, and of course physiology and anatomy has changed. Grant funding bodies are starting to recognise that people may take career breaks including parental leave and undertaking blind reviewing of grants, more journals are trying to combat unconscious bias in all areas by conducting blind reviews of papers, many institutions across the world have, or are implementing equality charters.

Evidently, women may still face challenges with regards to unequal pay, gaining leadership roles, recognition within their fields and even in many parts of the world being able to achieve an education which allows them to succeed. A similar situation can be observed for many men of course. However, there has been considerable progression for women in the field of sciences since the 1900s so hopefully these issues will be overcome in future years.

This book contains anatomical and physiological reviews and original research from across the world. Perhaps one of the greatest strengths of veterinary anatomy and physiology is the diverse research which we see from all over the world. This book contains work in a variety of species including the horse, dog, cattle and chickens. It covers areas such as the heart, tendons, prostate gland, and the hoof. In addition it covers not only normal anatomy and physiology but also diseases, disorders and blends in information for those in the veterinary professions.

Author details

Valentina Kubale[1], Emma Cousins[2], Clara Bailey[2], Samir A.A. El-Gendy[3] and Catrin Sian Rutland[2]*

1 Veterinary Faculty, University of Ljubljana, Ljubljana, Slovenia

2 School of Veterinary Medicine and Science, University of Nottingham, Nottingham, UK

3 Department of Anatomy and Embryology, Faculty of Veterinary Medicine, Alexandria University, Egypt

*Address all correspondence to: catrin.rutland@nottingham.ac.uk

References

[1] Clark W. A history of comparative anatomy. Nature. 1944;**154**:563

[2] Breasted. The Edwin Smith surgical papyrus. In: Facsimile and Hieroglyphic Transliteration with Translation and Commentary in Two Volumes. USA: The University of Chicago Oriental Institute Publications; 1930

[3] Cave AJ. Ancient Egypt and the origin of anatomical science. Proceedings of the Royal Society of Medicine. 1950;**43**(7):568-571

[4] Serageldin I. Ancient Alexandria and the dawn of medical science. Global Cardiology Science & Practice. 2013;**2013**(4):395-404

[5] Siddiquey AS, Husain SS, Laila SZH. History of anatomy. Bangladesh Journal of Anatomy. 2009;**7**(1):3

[6] Doty RW. Philosophy and the brain. Perspectives in Biology and Medicine. 1965;**9**(1):23-34

[7] Khan IA, Daya SK, Gowda RM. Evolution of the theory of circulation. International Journal of Cardiology. 2005;**98**(3):519-521

[8] Dobson JF. Herophilus of Alexandria. Proceedings of the Royal Society of Medicine. 1925;**18**(Sect Hist Med):19-32

[9] Crivellato E, Ribatti D. A portrait of Aristotle as an anatomist: Historical article. Clinical Anatomy (New York, NY). 2007;**20**(5):447-485

[10] Duckworth W. Galen on Anatomical Procedures: The Later Books. Cambridge: Cambridge University Press; 1962

[11] Toledo-Pereyra LH. Galen's contribution to surgery. Journal of the History of Medicine and Allied Sciences. 1973;**28**(4):357-375

[12] Pasipoularides A. Galen, father of systematic medicine. An essay on the evolution of modern medicine and cardiology. International Journal of Cardiology. 2014;**172**(1):47-58

[13] Nutton, Vivian. Early Modern/Renaissance Anatomy. In: eLS. Chichester: Sep 2015; John Wiley & Sons Ltd,. Available from: http://www.els.net. doi: 10.1002/9780470015902.a0025079]

[14] Olry R. Medieval neuroanatomy: The text of Mondino Dei Luzzi and the plates of guido da Vigevano. Journal of the History of the Neurosciences. 1997;**6**(2):113-123

[15] West JB. History of respiratory mechanics prior to World War II. Comprehensive Physiology. 2012;**2**(1):609-619

[16] Ribatti D. William Harvey and the discovery of the circulation of the blood. Journal of Angiogenesis Research. 2009;**1**:3

[17] Hutton F. The working of the 1832 Anatomy Act in Oxford and Manchester. Family & Community History. 2006;**9**(2):125-139

[18] McLachlan JC, Patten D. Anatomy teaching: Ghosts of the past, present and future. Medical Education. 2006;**40**(3):243-253

[19] Turney BW. Anatomy in a modern medical curriculum. Annals of the Royal College of Surgeons of England. 2007;**89**(2):104-107

[20] Murgitroyd E, Madurska M, Gonzalez J, Watson A. 3D digital anatomy modelling—Practical or pretty? The Surgeon: Journal of the Royal Colleges of Surgeons of Edinburgh and Ireland. 2015;**13**(3):177-180

[21] Araki T. The history of optical microscope. Mechanical Engineering Revision. 2017;**4**(1):16-00242. Available from: https://doi.org/10.1299/mer.16-00242

[22] Scatliff JH, Morris PJ. From Roentgen to magnetic resonance imaging: The history of medical imaging. North Carolina Medical Journal. 2014;**75**(2):111-113

[23] Chew FS, Relyea-Chew A, Ochoa ER Jr. Postmortem computed tomography of cadavers embalmed for use in teaching gross anatomy. Journal of Computer Assisted Tomography. 2006;**30**(6):949-954

[24] Dunn PM. Wilhelm Conrad Roentgen (1845-1923), the discovery of X-rays and perinatal diagnosis. Archives of Disease in Childhood Fetal and Neonatal Edition. 2001;**84**(2):F138-F139

[25] Reed AB. The history of radiation use in medicine. Journal of Vascular Surgery. 2011;**53**(1 Suppl):3s-5s

[26] Bhattacharyya KB. Godfrey Newbold Hounsfield (1919-2004): The man who revolutionized neuroimaging. Annals of Indian Academy of Neurology. 2016;**19**(4):448-450

[27] Ambrose J. CT scanning: A backward look. Seminars in Roentgenology. 1977;**12**(1):7-11

[28] Hounsfield GN. Computed medical imaging. Medical Physics. 1980;**7**(4):283-290. DOI:10.1118/1.594709

[29] Beckmann EC. CT scanning the early days. The British Journal of Radiology. 2006;**79**(937):5-8

[30] Campbell S. A short history of sonography in obstetrics and gynaecology. Facts, Views & Vision in ObGyn. 2013;**5**(3):213-229

[31] Provost J, Papadacci C, Arango JE, Imbault M, Fink M, Gennisson JL, et al. 3D ultrafast ultrasound imaging in vivo. Physics in Medicine and Biology. 2014;**59**(19):L1-Ll13

[32] Kurjak A. Ultrasound scanning—Prof. Ian Donald (1910-1987). European Journal of Obstetrics and Gynecology and Reproductive Biology. 2000;**90**(2):187-189

[33] Slavkovsky P, Uhliar R. The Nobel Prize in Physiology or Medicine in 2003 to Paul C. Lauterbur, Peter Mansfield for magnetic resonance imaging. Bratislavske Lekarske Listy. 2004;**105**(7-8):245-249

[34] Cammoun D, Hendee WR, Davis KA. Clinical applications of magnetic resonance imaging—Current status. The Western Journal of Medicine. 1985;**143**(6):793-803

[35] Watrous JD, Alexandrov T, Dorrestein PC. The evolving field of imaging mass spectrometry and its impact on future biological research. Journal of Mass Spectrometry. 2011;**46**(2):209-222

[36] Caprioli RM, Farmer TB, Gile J. Molecular imaging of biological samples: Localization of peptides and proteins using MALDI-TOF MS. Analytical Chemistry. 1997;**69**(23):4751-4760

[37] Gagnon H, Franck J, Wisztorski M, Day R, Fournier I, Salzet M. Targeted mass spectrometry imaging: Specific targeting mass spectrometry imaging technologies from history to perspective. Progress in Histochemistry and Cytochemistry. 2012;**47**(3):133-174

[38] Maidment AD. The future of medical imaging. Radiation Protection Dosimetry. 2010;**139**(1-3):3-7

[39] Keane M, Paul E, Sturrock CJ, Rauch C, Rutland CS. Computed tomography

in veterinary medicine: Currently published and tomorrow's vision. In: Halefoglu AM, editor. Computed Tomography: Advanced Applications. UK: IntechOpen; 2017. DOI: 10.5772/intechopen.68556

[40] Barber-Lomax JW, Bourgelat C. Journal of Small Animal Practice. 1964;**5**(1):3-4

[41] Pugh LP. The evolution of the veterinary profession in Great Britain. The British Veterinary Journal. 1967;**123**(10):423-430

[42] Bols PEJ, De Porte HFM. The horse catalyzed birth of modern veterinary medicine in 18th-century France. Journal of Equine Veterinary Science. 2016;**41**:35-41

[43] Irvine L, Vermilya JR. Gender work in a feminized profession: The case of veterinary medicine. Gender & Society. 2010;**24**(1):56-82

[44] Caple I. A short history of veterinary education in Australia: The 120-year transition from education for a trade to education for a profession. Australian Veterinary Journal. 2011;**89**(8):282-288

[45] Edwards JT. History of the veterinary profession 1851-1951: (a) The year 1881 as a great landmark in the modern history of the British veterinary profession the chief leaders in successful reform, with particular reference to John Henry steel. British Veterinary Journal. 1951;**107**(12):475 6.e1,7-6,6.e1,84

[46] Smith DF. Lessons of history in veterinary medicine. Journal of Veterinary Medical Education. 2013;**40**(1):2-11

[47] Smith DF. 150th anniversary of veterinary education and the veterinary profession in North America: Part 2, 1940-1970. Journal of Veterinary Medical Education. 2011;**38**(1):84-99

[48] Hall SA. Aleen Cust, Veterinary surgeon. Britain's first woman vet: Connie M. Ford The Orchard, Clanage Road, Bristol BS3 2JX: Biopress Ltd. 1990. 109 p. £5.99 (incl. p & p from publisher). British Veterinary Journal. 1991;**147**(5):486-487

[49] Boden E. Brancker (Winifred) Mary (1914-2010), Veterinary Surgeon. UK: Oxford University Press; 2014

[50] BVA. BVA_Presidents_1881_to_2013. 2018. Available from: https://www.bva.co.uk/uploadedFiles/Content/About_BVA/BVA_Presidents_1881_to_2013.pdf. [Accessed 07/08/2018]

[51] Crispin S, Clark JM. Uvarov, Dame Olga Nikolaevna (1910-2001), veterinary scientist. UK: Oxford University Press; 2005

[52] Allen LCV. Feminisation: Threat or opportunity? Veterinary Record. 2016;**178**(16):391-393

[53] Slater MR, Slater M. Women in veterinary medicine. Journal of the American Veterinary Medical Association. 2000;**217**(4):472

[54] RCVS. The UK veterinary profession in 2006: The findings of a survey of the profession conducted by the Royal College of veterinary surgeons. 2006. Available from: https://www.rcvs.org.uk/news-and-views/publications/rcvs-survey-of-the-professions-2006/surveyprofession2006.pdf. [Accessed 09/09/2018]

[55] RCVS. Women in the veterinary profession 2014: Gender statistics about veterinary surgeons in the UK. VetFutures. 2014. Available from: http://vetfutures.org.uk/download/factsheets/Gender%20statistics%20about%20veterinary%20surgeons%20in%20the%20UK.pdf. [Accessed 09/09/2018]

[56] Lincoln AE. The shifting supply of men and women to occupations: Feminization in veterinary education. Social Forces. 2010;**88**(5):1969-1998

[57] Lofstedt J. Gender and veterinary medicine. The Canadian Veterinary Journal = La revue veterinaire canadienne. 2003;**44**(7):533-535

[58] Drum S, Whiteley HE. Women in Veterinary Medicine: Profiles of Success. USA: Iowa State University Press; 1991

[59] AVMA. Market Research Statistics: U.S. Veterinarians 2017. 2017. Available from: https://www.avma.org/KB/Resources/Statistics/Pages/Market-research-statistics-US-veterinarians.aspx. [Accessed 08/09/2018]

[60] CVMA. Veterinary Demographics (2017). 2017. Available from: https://www.canadianveterinarians.net/about/statistics. [Accessed 07/09/2018]

[61] Prescott JF, Bailey J, Hagele WC, Leung D, Lofstedt J, Radostits OM, et al. CVMA task force on education, licensing, and the expanding scope of veterinary practice. The Canadian Veterinary Journal. 2002;**43**(11):845-854

[62] Gul RT, Ozkul T, Akcay A, Ozen A. Historical profile of gender in Turkish veterinary education. Journal of veterinary medical education. 2008;**35**(2):305-309

[63] Rezai-Rashti G, Moghadam V. Women and higher education in Iran: What are the implications for employment and the "marriage market"? International Review of Education. 2011;**57**(3-4):419-441

[64] Shepherd AJ, Pikel L. Employment of female and male graduates of us veterinary medical colleges, 2013. Journal of the American Veterinary Medical Association. 2013;**243**(8):1122-1126

[65] Honey L. Women as veterinary leaders and entrepreneurs. Veterinary Record. 2014;**175**(23):578

[66] RCVS. The 2014 RCVS Survey of the Veterinary Profession. 2014. Available from: https://www.rcvs.org.uk/news-and-views/publications/rcvs-survey-of-the-veterinary-profession-2014/rcvs-survey-of-the-veterinary-profession-2014.pdf. [Accessed 07/08/2018]

[67] Heath TJ. Longitudinal study of veterinary students and veterinarians: The first 20 years. Australian Veterinary Journal. 2007;**85**(7):281-289

[68] Smith CA. The gender shift in veterinary medicine: Cause and effect. Veterinary clinics of North America. Small Animal Practice. 2006;**36**(2):329-339

[69] Castro SM, Armitage-Chan E. Career aspiration in UK veterinary students: The influences of gender, self-esteem and year of study. Veterinary Record. 2016;**179**(16):408

[70] Alibhai A, Saiger MM, Harding E, Rutland CS. Is your extra X chromosome holding you Back? An insight into female education and academic careers in STEMM. In: New Pedagogical Challenges in the 21st Century [Internet]. UK: IntechOpen; 2018. pp. 251-267. Available from: https://www.intechopen.com/books/new-pedagogical-challenges-in-the-21st-century-contributions-of-research-in-education/is-your-extra-x-chromosome-holding-you-back-an-insight-into-female-education-and-academic-careers-in. DOI: 10.5772/intechopen.71898

[71] Wikipedia. Category: Women Anatomists. 2018. Available from: https://en.wikipedia.org/wiki/Category:Women_anatomists [cited: Nov 2, 2018]

DOI: http://dx.doi.org/10.5772/intechopen.82412

[72] Wikipedia. Alessandra Giliani. 2018. Available from: https://en.wikipedia.org/wiki/Alessandra_Giliani [cited: Nov 1, 2018]

[73] Wikipedia. Anna Morandi Manzolini. 2018. Available from: https://en.wikipedia.org/wiki/Anna_Morandi_Manzolini

[74] Wikipedia. Marion Bidder. 2018. Available from: https://en.wikipedia.org/wiki/Marion_Bidder

[75] Wikipedia. Vera Danchakoff. 2018. Available from: https://en.wikipedia.org/wiki/Vera_Danchakoff [cited: Nov 2, 2018]

[76] Wikipedia. Katharine Bishop. 2018. Available from: https://en.wikipedia.org/wiki/Katharine_Bishop

[77] Wikipedia. Ruth Bowden. 2018. Available from: https://en.wikipedia.org/wiki/Ruth_Bowden [cited: Nov 2, 2018]

[78] Wikipedia. Marian Diamond. 2018. Available from: https://en.wikipedia.org/wiki/Marian_Diamond [cited: Nov 2, 2018]

[79] Wilkipedia. Mary Anne Frey. 2018. Available from: https://en.wikipedia.org/wiki/Mary_Anne_Frey [cited Oct 1 2018]

[80] NobelMediaAB. Nobel Prize Awarded Women. 2018. Available from: https://www.nobelprize.org/prizes/lists/nobel-prize-awarded-women-3/ [cited oct 2 2018]

[81] WAVA. World Association of Veterinary Anatomists. 2018. Available from: http://www.wava-amav.org/ [cited Nov 2 2018]

[82] EAVA. European Association of Veterinary Anatomists. 2018 Available from: http://www.eava.eu.com/ [cited nov 2 2018]

[83] AAVA. American Association of Veterinary Anatomists. 2018. Available from: https://vetanatomists.org/ [cited nov 2 2018]

[84] AfricanAVA. African Association of Veterinary Anatomists. 2018. Available from: http://www.vetanat.com/Association-Society.htm [cited nov 2 2018]

[85] IUSP. International Union of Physiological Sciences. 2018. Available from: http://www.iups.org/ [cited nov 2 2018]

[86] FEPS. Federation of European Physiological Societies. 2018. Available from: http://www.feps.org/index.php [cited: Nov 2, 2018]

[87] APS. American Physiology Society. 2018. Available from: http://www.the-aps.org/ [cited: Nov 2, 2018]

[88] AAPS. African Association of Physiological Sciences. 2018. Available from: https://aapsnet.org/

[89] FAOPS. Federation of the Asian and Oceanian Physiological Societies. 2018. Available from: http://faops.org.my/ [cited: Nov 2, 2018]

Section 2

The Hoof and Musculoskeletal System

Chapter 2

The Anatomy, Histology and Physiology of the Healthy and Lame Equine Hoof

Ramzi Al-Agele, Emily Paul, Valentina Kubale Dvojmoc, Craig J. Sturrock, Cyril Rauch and Catrin Sian Rutland

Abstract

Satisfactory investigations of the equine foot appear to be limited by the histomorphological complexity of internal hoof structures. Foot lameness is considered to be one of the most debilitating pathological disorders of the equine foot. In most species, foot lameness is traditionally linked to hoof deformity, and a set of molecular events have been defined in relation to the disease. So far, there is controversy regarding the incidence of foot lameness in horses, as it is unclear whether it is foot lameness that triggers hoof distortions or vice-versa. In order to develop a better understanding of foot lameness, we review both the healthy and lame foot anatomy, cell biology and vascularisation and using micro-computed tomography show new methods of visualising internal structures within the equine foot.

Keywords: equine, anatomy, histology, healthy, lame, vasculature

1. Introduction

Understanding the basic anatomy of the horse hoof is essential in order to further investigate the structures' involvement in the pathogenesis of lameness and in order to help understand disorders such as lameness and laminitis. This chapter aims to show anatomy and physiology of the hoof and bones of the equine foot and relate these back to lameness and laminitis in the horse.

2. Gross anatomy of the equine hoof

The distal extremities of the domestic mammal are encased inside a keratinised capsule [1], which takes the form of a hoof capsule in ungulates and a claw in carnivores [2]. This insensitive horny structure encloses the distal part of the second phalanx (also known as the middle phalanx or short pastern bone), the distal phalanx (also known as the coffin bone or the pedal bone) and the navicular bone, in addition to connective tissues including, for example, the distal interphalangeal joint, medial and lateral hoof cartilage, with the terminal end of the deep digital flexor tendon and navicular bursa [1, 3–5]. These structures are connected to each other in order to provide a coherent and resilient structure within the foot (**Figure 1**) [6].

IntechOpen

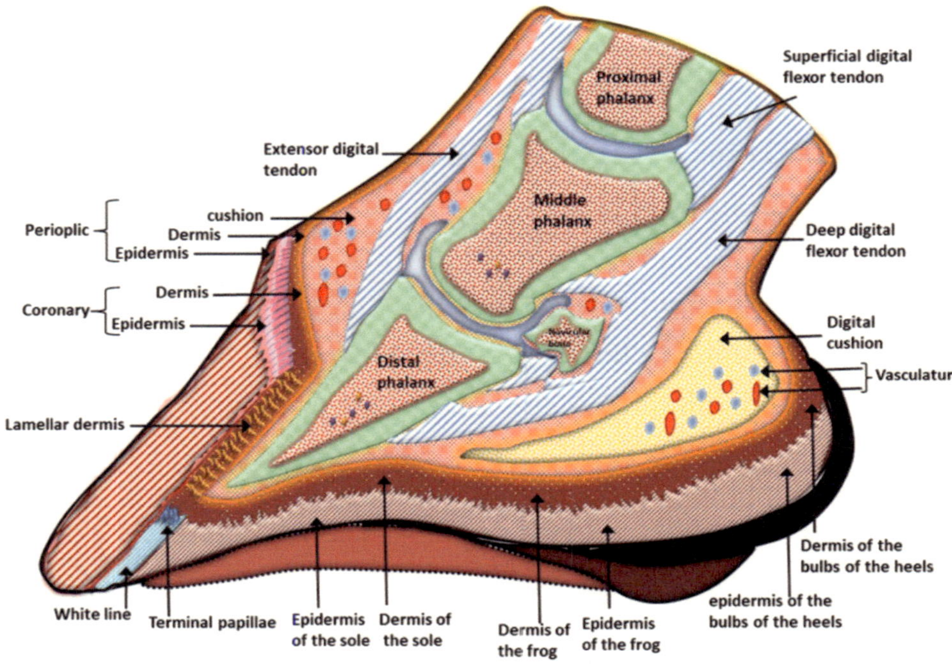

Figure 1.
Schematic drawing of a sagittal section of equine hoof. Schematic diagram illustrating the entire structure of the horse hoof. Figure adapted from Budras et al., [7].

The hoof is composed of horn, derived from epidermal tissue which has been keratinised to a varying extent [8]. Horn is largely arranged into a series of parallel microscopic tubules, interconnected by intertubular horn [9]. This structure plays a substantial role in load-bearing, and encapsulates almost the entire circumference of the foot, curling inwards towards the rear to form the bars which provide additional support to the heels [10]. Encasing the palmar/plantar surface of the foot is the sole, which is concave and has a similar, but softer and more flexible, composition to the hoof wall [10]. The hoof joins to the skin at the coronet where it is protected by a waterproof band of soft tubular horn, the periople [11]. Connecting the periphery of the sole to the hoof wall is the white line, which is highly elastic and derived from the epidermal lamellae. Composed of supple, incompletely keratinised horn, the frog is an elastic structure which is essential for shock absorption, blood circulation, and in slip prevention [10]. The frog extends inwards to the digital cushion which, being composed of poorly vascularised adipose tissue embedded in a fibroelastic mesh, is involved in shock absorbance and possesses blood pumping properties [6, 10]. The digital cushion is segregated from the deep digital flexor tendon (DDFT) by the presence of the distal digital annular ligament [10].

The bones of the equine foot comprise the third phalanx (P3; also called the distal phalanx), the second phalanx (P2), and the navicular bone. P3, also referred to as the pedal or coffin bone, is the foot's principal bone, occupying its most distal position, and attaching to the hoof capsule via the lamellar and solar coria [6]. P3 supports and stabilises the hoof capsule, and is highly porous due to the prolificacy of nutrient foramina [6]. P2, or short pastern, forms the proximal interphalangeal, or pastern, joint with the first phalanx (P1), and the distal interphalangeal, or coffin, joint with P3 [10]. Its short, nearly cuboidal, composure makes P2 resilient to a broad range of stresses [6]. The navicular, or distal sesamoid bone, is a small, smooth bone located caudal to the distal interphalangeal joint. Coated ventrally in smooth fibrocartilage, it has a pulley-like role, allowing the DDFT to glide smoothly under the distal interphalangeal joint without interference from other bones [10]. The navicular synovial bursa and distal synovial sheathes further aid the smooth action of the DDFT as it secretes synovial fluid which lubricates the area [10].

Along with the DDFT, which descends from the deep digital flexor muscle in the forearm to the flexor surface of P3, the superficial digital flexor tendon (SDFT) forms part of the back tendon pair, thus enabling flexion of the interphalangeal joints [10, 11]. Descending from the superficial digital flexor muscle in the forearm, the SDFT attaches to the proximal surfaces of P1 and P2 [10]. Responsible for the extension of the interphalangeal joints is the common digital extensor tendon (CDET also known as m. extensor digitorum communis in the fore limb and m. extensor digitorum longus on the rear limb) [11]. Stemming from the long digital extensor muscle proximal to the knee, the CDET descends the leg dorsally, terminating at the extensor process of P3 with projections into P1 and P2 [10].

While the DDFT and SDFT permit flexion of the foot's interphalangeal joints and the CDET allows their extension, the presence of lateral and medial collateral ligaments limits the joints' adduction and abduction respectively [11]. The collateral ligaments attach to notches on the distal and proximal edges of P1 and P2 correspondingly in the case of those of the proximal interphalangeal joint, and on the distal and proximal edges of P2 and P3 respectively for those of the distal interphalangeal joint [11]. The position of P3 is also maintained by three pairs of chondral ligaments, attaching to the medial and lateral cartilages of P3 [10]. The navicular bone is held in place by the navicular suspensory ligaments which anchor to the distal edge of P1, just dorsal to the collateral ligament attachments, and converge at the navicular bone, forming the distal navicular ligament which terminates at P3 [10].

The coria are the richly vascularised and innervated dermal regions lying between and supporting the skeletal structures and the epidermal hoof capsule [4]. The coronary corium runs along the proximal edge of the hoof wall, with each hoof wall tubule growing around small, finger-like papillae projecting from the coronary corium which provide nourishment to the proliferative epidermal cells, maintaining hoof growth [8]. The solar corium is similar in structure and function to the coronary corium, with papillae enabling the growth of the sole [8]. The lamellae of the lamellar corium, commonly referred to as the sensitive or the dermal lamellae, form, together with the epidermal/insensitive lamellae of the inner hoof wall with which they interlock, the suspensory apparatus of the third phalanx, suspending P3 within the hoof capsule [4]. Distal to each dermal lamella is a set of papillae, the terminal papillae, which form the soft, elastic white line which binds wall to sole [8].

The macroscopic ridge-like primary lamellae, of which there are some 550–600 epidermal/dermal interlocking pairs in parallel descent within each foot, provide a large surface area between the epidermis and the dermis for the suspension of P3 [9]. Each primary lamella bears a further 150–200 microscopic secondary lamellae and, collectively, the primary and secondary lamellae create a surface area for attachment of around 0.8 m^2 (**Figure 2**) [9].

Between the dermal and epidermal tissues of the foot lies the basement membrane (BM), a strong, uninterrupted sheet of extracellular matrix [8]. Epidermal basal cells are attached to the basement membrane (BM) on its border with the hoof epidermis [8]. On its inner, dermis-bordering side, a vast array of collagen-rich connective tissue strands projecting from the periosteum of P3 intertwine with the BM's lattice, ensuring the structural integrity of the dermal structures [8]. The BM is folded into ridges along the longitudinal axes of the primary lamellae, forming the secondary lamellae, and the coronary and terminal papillae, increasing the surface area for the attachment of proliferative epidermal basal cells [12].

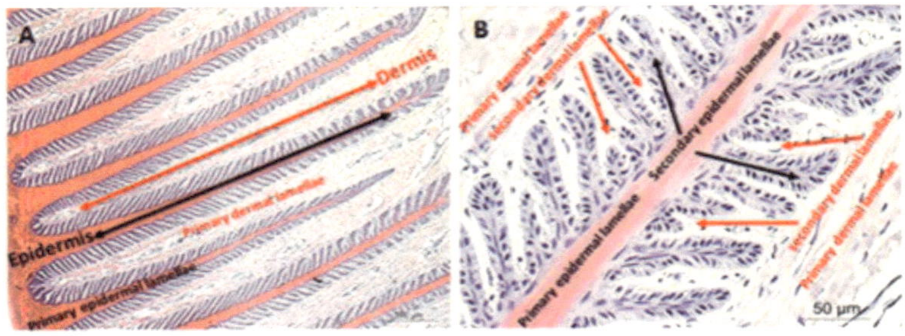

Figure 2.
Haematoxylin and eosin stained lamellae within the horse hoof.

3. Vasculature of the foot

In addition to the bones, ligaments, tendons and other soft tissues of the foot, the vasculature is essential in the equine foot. The blood vessel system is a vital part of transport of dissolved gases, nutrients, waste, signalling chemicals such as hormones, and immune cells to and from other organs [13]. The vast vascular network underlying the hoof capsule and coursing through the bones, fed through branches from the medial and lateral digital arteries and returning to general circulation via the medial and lateral digital veins (**Figure 3**) [9].

The vascular blood supply of the hoof originates from the common palmar digital artery and the dorsometatarsal artery, these main branches giving rise to medial and lateral palmar/plantar digital arteries (**Figure 4**) [14, 15]. In the hind limb, the small plantar common digital arteries contribute to form the digital arteries. At the level of second phalanx, there are branches nourishing to the heel bulbs and coronary region [1].

The vascular arteries of the dermis are divided into three independent arterial blood supplies: the dorsal coronary corium; the palmar/plantar portion of the coronary corium and laminar corium; and the dorsal laminar corium and solar corium, as the blood flow is reversely directed from the distal part to the proximal part within the dermal lamina (also termed lamella/lamellae and lamellar in the

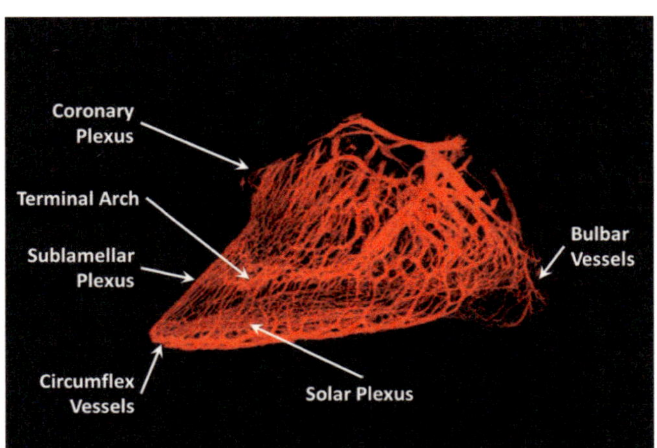

Figure 3.
Vascularisation of the equine foot. Reconstruction of the vasculature of the equine foot from CT images, showing the coronary, sublamellar and solar plexuses, the terminal arch, the circumflex vessels of the sole, and the bulbar vessels.

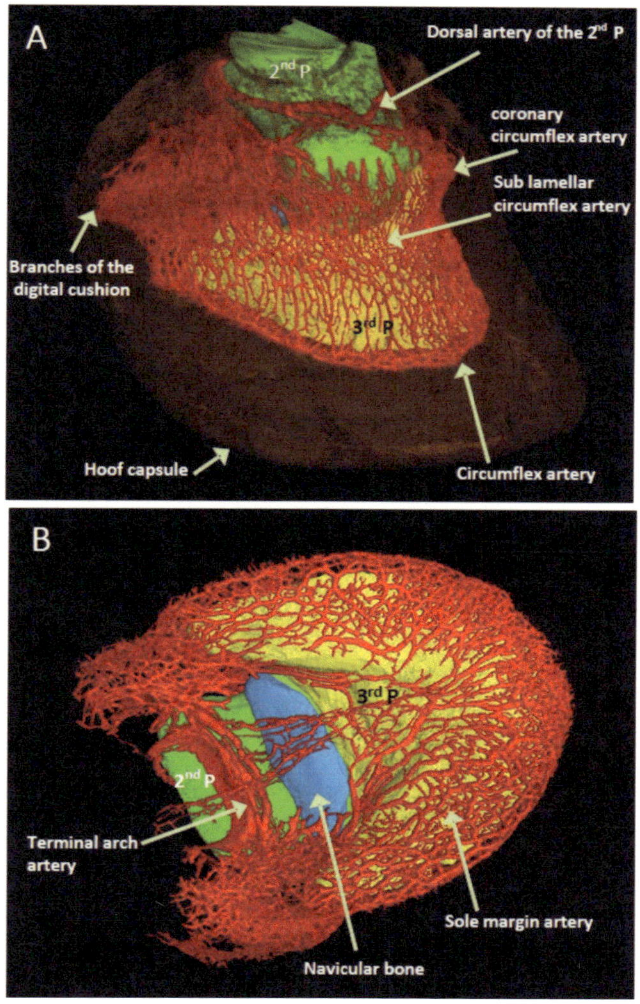

Figure 4.
Reconstruction of micro CT image illustrating vascularisation of equine foot. Computed tomography (CT) scan images showing the three-dimensional reconstruction of arterial supply of equine foot. (A) Shows arteries distributed throughout the dorsal surface of the distal phalanx and anastomoses located proximally with vessels of the coronet and distally forming the circumflex artery. (B) Represents the arteries distributed in the sole margin.

literature) [4]. The terminal branches of the blood supply enter the distal phalanx from the medial and lateral aspects and then form several anastomoses within the bone to make the terminal arch. At this arch, there are 8–10 blood vessels emerging distally to nourish the sole margin [1]. This is a highly important organisation of blood vessels in equine feet as the terminal arch and its branches are protected by the bony canal that can be altered in chronic laminitis, leading to ischemia and a decrease in the growth rate of the corium [16].

The capillary network of the equine digit is complex due to the fact that the dorsal and palmar parts of the foot have different blood supplies and drainage routes [2]. For instance, the blood vessels of the dorsal lamella pass through the distal phalanx and the blood supply of these portions is directed in the distal to the proximal way, while the palmar lamella is from the proximal circumflex to dorsal lamella [17]. Thus, haemorrhage from the sublamellar circulation can result in the rotation of P3, as is observed in the case of founder [16, 18, 19]. Consequently, the blood vessels of the equine foot are predisposed to local vasoconstriction and the development of ischemic disease as the arteries from the plexus have thicker walls with small lumens and are unable to auto-regulate the volume variations that are involved in contraction of smooth muscle as well as encompassing arteriovenous shunts [18].

The equine hoof veins are divided into three groups depending on their location: wall dermis veins, which are separated into proximal and distal regions; coronary dermis veins; and frog and sole dermis veins [1]. The dermal lamella is drained by: the coronary vein; the independent superficial vein; the proximal branch of the caudal hoof vein; and the circumflex vein. The toe and quarters are drained via the circumflex vein [2, 20]. An additional feature of the blood circulation of the equine foot is the anastomoses of arteries and veins, which are blood vessels forming shunts [21]. Each dermal papilla in the periople, coronary band, frog, sole and terminal papillae contain a meshwork of anastomosing arteriovenous vessels located at the base of the papillae. These anastomoses are able to withdraw approximately 50% of the whole limb blood flow, and thus can be involved in ischemia due to blood flow diversion [22]. This could explain the relationship between laminitis and ischemia [3].

4. Bone physiology

Bone is a complex, dynamic tissue that has the ability to grow ontogenically, to repair after damage, and to adaptively respond to a variety of exogenous and endogenous stimuli [23]. Composed of a mineralised organic matrix in which the cells responsible for its formation and rejuvenation are embedded, osseous tissue, through its unique physiological and biochemical properties, enables bones to perform a multitude of functions within the animal's body. The organic matrix, or osteoid [24], is formed principally of type-I collagen (around ~95% type-I [25]) which affords the bone its tensile strength, alongside trace amounts of other collagens, in addition to non-collagenous proteins whose predominant purpose is to permit the mineralisation of the matrix. The chief mineral salt found in osseous tissue is a form of hydroxyapatite [$Ca_{10}(PO_4)_6(OH)_2$] which, bound to the matrix proteins, renders the tissue resistant to compressive forces [23].

The bone is structured into either cortical or trabecular bone. Cortical, or compact, bone forms the dense outer proportions of the bone and, in the human, accounts for 80% of the total skeletal mass [23, 26]. Cortical osteons (**Figure 5**), or Haversian systems, are tubular structures consisting of a central channel (Haversian canal), through which a nerve and blood supply are provided,

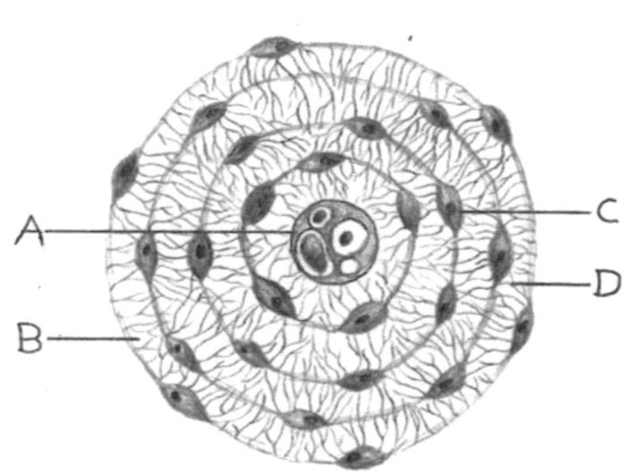

Figure 5.
Schematic of a cortical osteon. (A) Represents a Haversian canal incorporating a neurovascular bundle, (B) a lamella, (C) a lacuna containing an osteocyte, and (D) canaliculi.

surrounded by coaxial lamellae of mineralised bone matrix which incorporate a number of voids, in the form of lacunae and canaliculi, inhabited by cells [23]. The remaining 20% of the osseous tissue is in the form of trabeculae (from the Latin *trabs*, meaning "beam" [27]) which provide structural support, in a buttress-like manner, to the surrounding cortex. Trabecular osteons, or packets, are similar in their lamellar architecture to those of the cortex, but are smaller in size and semi-lunar in shape [23]. This hierarchical design, a common (if not omni-existent) phenomenon in biological materials, provides bones with the physical strength they need to fulfil their roles in structural support, the protection of underlying organs, and in providing leverage to muscles and tendons, facilitating movement [23, 28, 29].

The remodelling and general renewal of the bone is mediated by three cell types: osteoblasts, osteoclasts and osteocytes [30]. Osteoblasts are mononucleated cells formed by the differentiation of mesenchymal stem cells, and are responsible for the synthesis of osteoid and its subsequent mineralisation [25]. They reside principally in the endosteum—the vascularised cellular lining of the internal proportions of the bone, covering the walls of the Haversian canals, and the trabeculae and medullary cavity where it separates the bone matrix from the marrow [31]—and, alongside their incompletely-differentiated precursors and fibroblasts, the cambial layer of the periosteum [23]—a vascularised and innervated structure consisting of an outer fibrous layer comprising fibroblasts, collagen and elastin, and the discrete inner cambium that coats the bone's exterior [32]. Osteoclasts are multinucleated macrophagic cells derived from phagocytes in the haematopoietic bone marrow, and carry out bone resorption in localised areas of the bone surface to which they adhere upon activation [21]. Osteocytes, which inhabit the lacunae of the osteons and have multiple cytoplasmic processes which traverse the osteons' canaliculi, are the result of the terminal differentiation of osteoblasts that have become entrapped within the bone matrix that they have synthesised [25]. They act as mechanoreceptors, communicating with the osteogenic/osteolytic cells via gap junctions at the extremities of their cytoplasmic processes, and play a regulatory role in the bone synthesis/resorption cycle [25].

Concomitant to the physical need for the bone to be able to remodel for general maintenance, repair, and for increasing structural strength in response to stimuli, are the roles in pH balance and mineral homeostasis that the synthesis/resorption cycle affords [23]. While under normal physiological circumstances the pH of blood and extracellular fluid is maintained within narrow parameters by the removal and excretion of protons by the kidneys and lungs, a multitude of physiologically adverse conditions (e.g. kidney disease or severe exercise) can lead to acidosis [33]. The basicity of hydroxyapatite renders bone an emergency reservoir for base, buffering the acidity with the products of osteoclastic resorption. This mechanism is enabled by the osteoclast's stimulation at low pH, a peculiarity from a general cellular point of view, and the osteoblast's synergistic inhibition [33]. In a similar vein, bone acts as a reservoir for calcium and phosphorus, making them available for the maintenance of mineral homeostasis. Calcium and phosphorus are vital for a plethora of biological functions, and their homeostasis is under the endocrine regulation of the parathyroid glands, thyroid gland, and the kidney which, through the intermediary of parathyroid hormone, calcitriol (1,25-dihydroxyvitamin D, a hormone derived from vitamin D), and calcitonin respectively, affect the intestinal absorption, renal reabsorption and bone synthesis/resorption mechanisms [24, 34]. The parathyroid glands, which express Ca^{2+}-sensing receptors, secrete PTH in response to a reduction in circulating calcium ions. Parathyroid hormone acts in the kidney to decrease phosphate and increase calcium reabsorption, and in the bone by stimulating osteocytic and osteoclastic activity [34].

Bone also acts as reservoir for growth factors and cytokines, which are released during bone resorption and take effect either locally or systemically [14]. Along with the effects that these growth factors and cytokines may exert on other tissue cell types, such as the endothelial cells of the vasculature, they play important roles in bone formation and resorption, including: insulin-like growth factors, transforming growth factors, and bone morphogenic proteins as growth factors promoting osteogenesis; epidermal growth factor, granulocyte-macrophage colony-stimulating factor, macrophage-colony stimulating factor, and tumour necrosis factor as growth factors stimulating osteolytic resorption; platelet-derived growth factor and fibroblastic growth factor which have contributory effects to both bone formation and resorption; prostaglandins and leukotrienes as osteolysis-stimulating cytokines; and interleukins that may directly or indirectly stimulate either bone formation or resorption depending on the interleukin family in question [35].

Strong links exist between the skeletal and vascular systems and, along with a strong vascular and nerve presence in the periosteum, numerous neurovascular bundles enter the bone through nutrient foramina, descend and ascend the canals of Haversian systems, and enter medullary cavity through Volkmann's Canals [36]. The two systems are interdependent in that the bone relies on the vasculature for the delivery of oxygen and nutrients and that, modulated by osteoblasts, haematopoiesis takes place in the bone marrow [37].

5. Morphological changes and pathologies in the foot

The external morphology of the hoof capsule is indirectly associated with the function and shape of the internal segments of the hoof [38]. Dyson and colleagues [39] drew attention to the fact that, despite differences in the orientation of the distal phalanx between horses, mainly associated with changes in direction of the dished solar border, the morphology of the distal phalanx is unaffected by the external features of the hoof capsule. It is worth noting here that hoof shape can be altered when trimming and shoeing are considered [40]. The impact of trimming/shoeing on the hoof capsule shape has been explained [41] and the researchers demonstrated that the formation of the hoof wall is physically connected to the loading of the lower limb, thus protecting its optimal balance on the ground [42]. Therefore, the geometrical tendency of the foot components determines the ability of the internal structures to respond to loading through the bearing phase of the stride cycle [43].

The distal phalanx is attached within the hoof capsule through the suspensory apparatus [44], which connects the entire parietal surface of the distal phalanx to the lamellar structures of the internal hoof wall [11]. Preliminary work on equine lamellar connection found that this attachment provides the mechanism by which the weight is transferred between the distal phalanx and the epidermal laminae of the hoof wall [45]. This connection, or attachment, has a substantial role in the biomechanics of healthy foot performance, and may lead to foot lameness if damaged [41]. Indeed, the failure of the connection between the epidermal laminae and the underlying basement membrane of the dermal lamellae would weaken the suspensory apparatus of the distal phalanx [46]. Unsurprisingly, changes in the basement membrane of the suspensory tissue have been suggested to signal the first step of laminar failure [47]. While other research reported that lesions in the basement membrane appear before any clinical signs of foot lameness [48]. The dislocation of the distal phalanx, followed by its rotation, applies pressure, first on the sole at the palmar border of the distal phalanx and, secondly, on the coronet or upper area of the lamellae by the extensor process of the distal phalanx [49]. These deflections lead to impaired blood flow into the basal layers of the hoof wall [18], and can lead to an inhibition of the growth rate of the hoof capsule, affecting its shape over time and induced osteolysis of bone trabeculae in chronic stages [50]. A number of hoof shapes can arise from this chronic condition, including sheared heels, crushed heels, club foot, long-dished toe, and high-heel foot [49, 51].

One of these chronic conditions is the lamellar wedge that develops alongside laminitis and a result can be an anatomical displacement of the distal phalanx within the hoof capsule [52], is a direct consequence of the failure of the suspensory apparatus of the distal phalanx [53]. However, the molecular events involved in the lamellar wedge condition are broadly unknown [54]. In chronically laminitic horses, the lamellar wedge appears as an abnormal horny mass, that is formed between the inner hoof wall and the epidermal lamellae, and is linked to the slight rotation of the distal phalanx [55]. The separation of the distal phalanx inside the capsular wall can change the sole shape to become convex rather than be concave, due to differential growth of the proximal hoof wall portion [55]. The structural and physical appearance of this abnormal keratinized material is comparable to the white line tissue, and is therefore proposed to be an ectopic white line [56]. It was therefore thought that a large quantity of the ectopic white line could be able ultimately to prohibit the straight and normal growth of the hoof capsule (**Figure 6**) [57].

5.1 Lameness

Foot lameness is a physical impairment of a limb that has a negative effect on the freedom of movement of the animal [58, 59]. It is accompanied by clinical signs linked to a disturbance of locomotion that is related to hoof pathologies that can be caused by infection, environmental and/or genetic causes [60, 61]. Lameness can also manifest itself in pain and lesions that, in turn, lead to an abnormal gait [62, 63] with undesirable consequences on performance [64] and welfare [65]. This disruption in gait originates from involuntary and voluntary exertions to diminish the level of discomfort and/or pain that are the result of damage or injury of ligaments, muscles, nerves or integument [59, 60], or could be due to asymmetric and/or uneven feet promoting the development of foot lameness [66].

Virtually all ungulate animals can be affected by foot lameness [67–70]. However, our knowledge concerning the aetiology of the condition is often related to the economic implications of the animal in our society [58, 62]. Foot lameness is classified into acute and chronic types depending on the severity of lesions and the

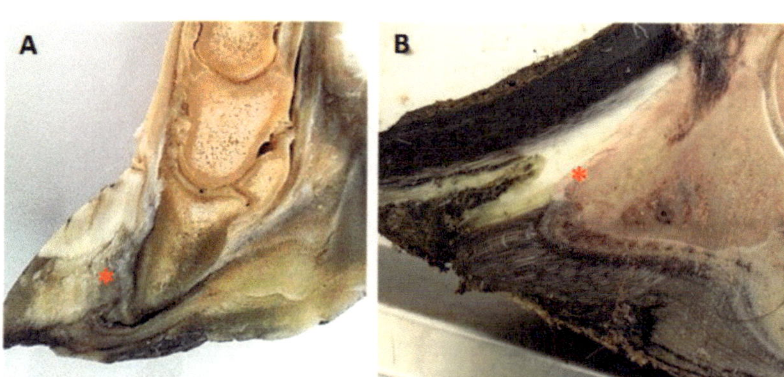

Figure 6.
*The anatomical displacement (indicated by *) of the distal phalanx. (A, B) Longitudinal section of two laminitic feet shows lamellae wedge inside the hoof capsule indicates (*) abnormal tissue, which changed the shape of hoof capsule.*

time requirement for healing, if healing is possible [71]. In dairy cows it represents the most important financial and welfare problem faced by the industry [60], as it is responsible for a drop in reproductive efficacy, a decrease in milk production, and increased culling rates [5, 69]. Similarly, in horses, foot lameness is a significant and predominant medical disorder which accounts for about to $1 billion in losses annually for the equine industry in the United States of America [72, 73]. In the UK, the maintenance of each horse is estimated to cost about £2660 annually and much of this in the treatment of foot lameness [74]. Foot lameness in the horse is the most prevalent and frequent medical issue, affecting about 11% of the general equine population in the UK in 2011 [75]. This rose significantly in 2012 to 18.6% [76] and was thought to be due to factors such as differing foot balance, shoeing and trimming techniques. Some subpopulations however, seem to be more affected than others as, for example, it is estimated that nearly 33% of dressage horses in the UK suffer from foot lameness [69]. The clinical diagnosis of foot lameness in the equine population is subdivided into scores ranging from 0 to 5 depending on the degree of the condition, with 5 being the worst outcome [77].

Lame horses adapt their gait to compensate for the pain originating from damaged tissues or foot lesions [78–80]. Accordingly, foot lameness is considered to be one of the most common signs of kinetic disorder affecting the musculoskeletal system [30]. As forelimb foot lameness is more common than hind limb foot lameness [81], it has been suggested that conformations of the distal limbs may have a substantial impact in the development of front and rear limb foot lameness [66]. The relatively high prevalence of forelimb foot lameness [81] which reaches to more than 75% of equine foot lameness being found in a forelimb particularly in breeds such as Thoroughbred horses and 40% in Standardbred racehorses [82]. This may be explained by that fact that the centre of gravity of the horse is closer to the front limbs than the rear limbs, as the loading ratio is spread approximately 60% forelimbs: 40% hind limbs [66]. Other research [80] has shown that horses with severe foot lameness in the front limb display an untrue foot lameness in the contralateral rear limb, whereas horses with a real rear limb foot lameness exhibit an incorrect foot lameness in the ipsilateral front limb.

Although the aetiology of equine foot lameness is still an active research area, recent efforts have also tried to determine whether the hoof shape is a disposing factor for foot lameness-causing lesions. The investigation of variations between foot lameness and non-foot lameness affected horses [51], demonstrated that the angle between the capsular wall and the ground is larger in the lame horse with an enlarged heel, curved or misshapen coronary band, that diverging growth lines can occur, and that the tubular horns differ from non-lame horses. It was suggested that hereditary influences and trimming are factors contributing to the asymmetrical shape of the hoof [83, 84].

In chronic foot lameness, the hoof capsule of the lame foot can be more distorted than in the non-lame one [85], as a result of altered loading forces applied to the hoof, hence affecting the shape of the hoof and the internal structures of the foot [86, 87]. These variations in the shape of the capsule are triggered by biological sources causing autolysis of the collagen fibres connecting the epithelium to the bone [68]. The role of these fibres is to support and suspend the weight of the horse via the distal phalanx, as well as to maintain the shape of the capsule constant [88, 89]. Another cause that could lead to hoof distortion is the ability of the foot to produce keratinous material proximally [90]. A number of chronic foot lameness states can be related to sheared heels causing palmar foot pain and hoof deviation [34]. Sheared heels are considered as one of the main causes of foot lameness in the equine genus, which results from an abnormal stride and persistent uneven weight bearing [91]. This leads to higher soft tissue strains that predispose the hoof capsule to deformation [92].

The hoof conformation seems to be a two-way process whereby the hoof shape is a key factor in foot lameness [54, 93] and foot deformation can arise as a consequence of foot lameness [85]. However, there has been little evidence showing that malformation is one of the predisposing factors for foot soreness and foot lameness. Dyson and colleagues [39] highlighted that, despite the differences in the shape of the distal phalanx between horses, lameness is mainly associated with changes in the direction of the dorsal hoof wall. For example, constant shoeing has an impact on the way in which the hoof grows and can, over time; result in a different foot conformation/capsular shape, which can have an effect on foot lameness [15, 40]. Recent bovine work using micro CT has shown that lame cows can present with additional bone growth on the distal phalanx [94]. It is important to remember that comparative findings in other animals could provide crucial evidence which may be applicable to horses and is therefore a further consideration for work in this area.

The methodologies which are used are also being developed over time and giving new insights into anatomy and physiology. In a recent study looking at foals with osteomyelitis it was shown how important newer techniques such as CT could be used to compliment traditional radiography whilst also providing novel information about disorders [95], the emerging evidence indicating that CT may be superior at detecting osseous changes in general in comparison to traditional techniques. The number of studies comparing MRI methods to more traditional methods is also highlighting the knowledge that can be gained in not only osseous tissue but also in soft tissue. For example in recent studies in equine limbs lesions where MRI was considered against retrospective patient data/ultrasonography radiography [96, 97]. In addition anatomical knowledge and imaging are becoming increasingly important for new discoveries and techniques in relation to stem cell and gene therapy as highlighted by recent studies using gene therapy to treat equine lameness [78, 98].

6. Conclusions

There is no doubt that understanding the anatomy, histology and physiology of the equine foot and limb is essential in treating a wide range of disorders. Advances in technology such as magnetic resonance imaging, computed tomography and other imaging techniques also play a role in assisting both anatomical knowledge and understanding equine conditions [99]. Coupled with more traditional techniques recent research has used these techniques to show bone conformation and growth, vascularisation and a number of other factors which could help inform us about anatomy and limb disorders. Although much is known about equine anatomy and histology, more is being discovered in both the normal and pathologically affected horse. In addition, new information from cellular and molecular studies is advancing not only the anatomical and histological sides but also the physiology and function of the equine limbs and the disorders they are prone to.

Acknowledgements

The work was funded by PetPlan, Waltham, The Ministry of Higher Education and Scientific Research of Iraq, Western Scholarship and The University of Nottingham School of veterinary Medicine and Science. We also thank Mr. Craig Sturrock CIPB, Hounsfield Building, University of Nottingham with whom the computed tomography imaging was carried out. Catrin Rutland Orcid: 0000-0002-2009-4898. Cyril Rauch Orcid: 0000-0001-8584-420X.F. Emily Paul Orcid: 0000-0001-8518-4205.

Conflict of interest

The authors declare no conflict of interest.

Nomenclature

Nomenclature observes Nomina Anatomica Veterinaria terminology [100].

Acronyms and abbreviations

BM	basement membrane
CDET	common digital extensor tendon
CT	computed tomography
DDFT	deep digital flexor tendon
P1	first phalanx
P2	second phalanx
P3	third phalanx
SDFT	superficial digital flexor tendon.

Author details

Ramzi Al-Agele[1,2], Emily Paul[1], Valentina Kubale Dvojmoc[3], Craig J. Sturrock[4], Cyril Rauch[1] and Catrin Sian Rutland[1]*

1 School of Veterinary Medicine and Science, University of Nottingham, Leicestershire, UK

2 Department of Anatomy, College of Veterinary Medicine, University of Diyala, Iraq

3 Veterinary Faculty, University of Ljubljana, Ljubljana, Slovenia

4 CPIB, The Hounsfield Facility, School of Biosciences, University of Nottingham, Leicestershire, UK

*Address all correspondence to: catrin.rutland@nottingham.ac.uk

References

[1] Bragulla H, Konig HE, Liebich H-G. Veterinary Anatomy of Domestic Mammals: Textbook and Colour Atlas. Germany: Schattauer Verlag; 2007

[2] Konig HE, Liebich H-G. Veterinary Anatomy of Domestic Mammals: Textbook and Color Atlas. Germany: Schattauer; 2007

[3] Stewart J. Understanding the Horse's Feet. UK: The Crowood Press; 2013

[4] Pollitt CC. The anatomy and physiology of the suspensory apparatus of the distal phalanx. Veterinary Clinics of North America: Equine Practice. 2010;**26**(1):29-49

[5] Budras KD, Sack WO. Anatomy of the Horse. UK: Manson Publishing; 2012

[6] Davies HMS, Philip CJ, Merritt JS. Functional anatomy of the equine digit: Determining function from structure. In: Floyd AE, Mansmann RA, editors. Equine Podiatry. Missouri: Saunders Elsevier; 2007

[7] Budras K-D, Sack WO, Rock S. Anatomy of the Horse: An Illustrated Text. Germany: Schlütersche; 2003

[8] Pollitt CC. Anatomy and physiology of the inner hoof wall. Clinical Techniques in Equine Practice. 2004;**3**(1):3-21

[9] Pollitt CC. Microscopic anatomy and physiology of the hoof. In: Floyd AE, Mansmann RA, editors. Equine Podiatry. Missouri: Saunders Elsevier; 2007. pp. 90-101

[10] Goody PC. Horse Anatomy: A Pictorial Approach to Equine Structure. 2nd ed. London: J. A. Allen; 2000

[11] Davies HMS, Philip C. Gross anatomy of the equine digit. In: Floyd AE, Mansmann RA, editors. Equine Podiatry. Missouri: Saunders Elsevier; 2007. pp. 1-24

[12] Pollitt CC. The basement membrane at the equine hoof dermal epidermal junction. Equine Veterinary Journal. 1994;**26**(5):399-407

[13] Stapor P, Wang X, Goveia J, Moens S, Carmeliet P. Angiogenesis revisited—role and therapeutic potential of targeting endothelial metabolism. Journal of Cell Science. 2014;**127**(Pt 20):4331-4341

[14] Delany AM, Canalis E. The metastasis-associated metalloproteinase stromelysin-3 is induced by transforming growth factor-beta in osteoblasts and fibroblasts. Endocrinology. 2001;**142**(4):1561-1566

[15] Baxter GM. Adams and Stashak's Foot Lameness in Horses. UK: John Wiley & Sons; 2011. pp. 516-520

[16] Floyd A, Mansmann R. Equine Podiatry. USA: Elsevier Health Sciences; 2007

[17] Collins JN, Galuppo LD, Thomas HL, Wisner ER, Hornof WJ. Use of computed tomography angiography to evaluate the vascular anatomy of the distal portion of the forelimb of horses. American Journal of Veterinary Research. 2004;**65**(10):1409-1420

[18] Hood DM, Grosenbaugh DA, Mostafa MB, Morgan SJ, Thomas BC. The role of vascular mechanisms in the development of acute equine laminitis. Journal of Veterinary Internal Medicine. 1993;**7**(4):228-234

[19] Orsini JA. A fresh look at the process of arriving at a clinical prognosis part 1: Laminitis. Journal of Equine Veterinary Science. 2011;**31**(4):194-201

[20] Mishra PC, Leach DH. Extrinsic and intrinsic veins of the equine Hoof wall. Journal of Anatomy. 1983;**136**:543-560

[21] Pearson OM, Lieberman DE. The aging of Wolff's "law": Ontogeny and responses to mechanical loading in cortical bone. American Journal of Physical Anthropology. 2004;**39**(Suppl):63-99

[22] Pollitt CC. The role of arteriovenous anastomoses in the pathophysiology of equine laminitis. In: Proceedings of the Thirty-Seventh Annual Convention of the American Association of Equine Practitioners. 1992. pp. 711-720

[23] Clarke B. Normal bone anatomy and physiology. Clinical Journal of the American Society of Nephrology. 2008;**3**(Suppl 3):S131-S139

[24] Petersen OH, editor. Lecture Notes on Human Physiology. 5th ed. Oxford: Blackwell Publishing; 2007

[25] Bayliss L, Mahoney DJ, Monk P. Normal bone physiology, remodelling and its hormonal regulation. Surgery (Oxford). 2012;**30**(2):47-53

[26] Iolascon G, Napolano R, Gioia M, Moretti A, Riccio I, Gimigliano F. The contribution of cortical and trabecular tissues to bone strength: Insights from denosumab studies. Clinical Cases in Mineral and Bone Metabolism : The Official Journal of the Italian Society of Osteoporosis, Mineral Metabolism, and Skeletal Diseases. 2013;**10**(1):47-51

[27] Stevenson A, Waite M, editors. Concise Oxford Dictionary. 12th ed. Oxford: Oxford University Press; 2011

[28] Gao HJ. Application of fracture mechanics concepts to hierarchical biomechanics of bone and bone-like materials. International Journal of Fracture. 2006;**138**(1-4):101-137

[29] Wegst UG, Bai H, Saiz E, Tomsia AP, Ritchie RO. Bioinspired structural materials. Nature Materials. 2015;**14**(1):23-36

[30] Nakahama K. Cellular communications in bone homeostasis and repair. Cellular and Molecular Life Sciences. 2010;**67**(23):4001-4009

[31] Pazzaglia UE, Congiu T, Sibilia V, Quacci D. Osteoblast-osteocyte transformation. A SEM densitometric analysis of endosteal apposition in rabbit femur. Journal of Anatomy. 2014;**224**(2):132-141

[32] Allen MR, Hock JM, Burr DB. Periosteum: Biology, regulation, and response to osteoporosis therapies. Bone. 2004;**35**(5):1003-1012

[33] Arnett T. Regulation of bone cell function by acid-base balance. Proceedings of the Nutrition Society. 2003;**62**(2):511-520

[34] Peacock M. Calcium metabolism in health and disease. Clinical Journal of the American Society of Nephrology. 2010;**5**(Suppl 1):S23-S30

[35] Kini U, Nandeesh BN. Physiology of bone formation, remodeling, and metabolism. In: Fogelman I, Gnanasegaran G, van der Wall H, editors. Radionuclide and Hybrid Bone Imaging. Berlin Heidelberg: Springer; 2012. pp. 29-57

[36] Stocum DL. Regenerative Biology and Medicine. 2nd ed. London: Elsevier; 2012

[37] Taichman RS. Blood and bone: Two tissues whose fates are intertwined to create the hematopoietic stem-cell niche. Blood. 2005;**105**(7):2631-2639

[38] Moleman M, Heel M, Weeren P, Back W. Hoof growth between two shoeing sessions leads to a substantial increase of the moment about the distal, but not the proximal, interphalangeal joint. Equine Veterinary Journal. 2006;**38**:170-174

[39] Dyson SJ, Tranquille CA, Collins SN, Parkin TDH, Murray RC. An

investigation of the relationships between angles and shapes of the hoof capsule and the distal phalanx. Equine Veterinary Journal. 2011;**43**(3):295-301

[40] van Heel MCV, van Weeren PR, Back W. Compensation for changes in hoof conformation between shoeing sessions through the adaptation of angular kinematics of the distal segments of the limbs of horses. American Journal of Veterinary Research. 2006;**67**(7):1199-1203

[41] Johnston C, Back W. Hoof ground interaction: When biomechanical stimuli challenge the tissues of the distal limb. Equine Veterinary Journal. 2006;**38**(7):634-641

[42] Ramsey G. Equine Hoof Biomechanics. New Zealand: The University of Auckland; 2011

[43] Gunnarsson V, Stefansdottir GJ, Jansson A, Roepstorff L. The effect of rider weight and additional weight in Icelandic horses in tolt: Part II. Stride parameters responses. Animal. 2017;**11**(9):1567-1572

[44] Pollitt C, Collins S. The suspensory apparatus of the distal phalanx in normal horses. Equine Veterinary Journal. 2016;**48**:496-501

[45] Douglas JE, Biddick TL, Thomason JJ, Jofriet JC. Stress/strain behaviour of the equine laminar junction. The Journal of Experimental Biology. 1998;**201**(15):2287-2297

[46] Eades SC. Overview of current laminitis research. Veterinary Clinics of North America: Equine Practice. 2010;**26**(1):51-63

[47] Visser MB, Pollitt CC. The timeline of lamellar basement membrane changes during equine laminitis development. Equine Veterinary Journal. 2011;**43**(4):471-477

[48] Kyaw-Tanner M, Pollitt CC. Equine laminitis: Increased transcription of matrix metalloproteinase-2 (MMP-2) occurs during the developmental phase. Equine Veterinary Journal. 2004;**36**(3):221-225

[49] Redden RF. Hoof capsule distortion: Understanding the mechanisms as a basis for rational management. Veterinary Clinics of North America: Equine Practice. 2003;**19**(2):443-462

[50] Engiles JB, Galantino-Homer HL, Boston R, McDonald D, Dishowitz M, Hankenson KD. Osteopathology in the equine distal phalanx associated with the development and progression of laminitis. Veterinary Pathology. 2015;**52**(5):928-944

[51] Dyson SJ, Tranquille CA, Collins SN, Parkin TDH, Murray RC. External characteristics of the lateral aspect of the hoof differ between non-lame and lame horses. Veterinary Journal. 2011;**190**(3):364-371

[52] Carter RA, Shekk V, de Laat MA, Pollitt CC, Galantino-Homer HL. Novel keratins identified by quantitative proteomic analysis as the major cytoskeletal proteins of equine (*Equus caballus*) hoof lamellar tissue. Journal of Animal Science. 2010;**88**(12):3843-3855

[53] Collins SN, van Eps AW, Pollitt CC, Kuwano A. The lamellar wedge. Veterinary Clinics of North America: Equine Practice. 2010;**26**(1):179-195

[54] Bragulla H, Hirschberg RM. Horse hooves and bird feathers: Two model systems for studying the structure and development of highly adapted integumentary accessory organs—The role of the dermo-epidermal interface for the micro-architecture of complex epidermal structures. Journal of Experimental Zoology Part B. 2003;**298b**(1):140-151

[55] Pollitt CC. Equine laminitis. Clinical Techniques in Equine Practice. 2004;**3**:34-44

[56] O'Grady SE. A fresh look at white line disease. Equine Veterinary Education. 2011;**23**(10):517-522

[57] Kuwano A, Katayama Y, Kasashima Y, Okada K, Reilly JD. A gross and histopathological study of an ectopic white line development in equine laminitis. The Journal of Veterinary Medical Science. 2002;**64**(10):893-900

[58] Archer S, Bell N, Huxley J. Foot lameness in UK dairy cows: A review of the current status. In Practice. 2010;**32**:492-504

[59] Animal WC. In: ACM MG, editor. Physiotherapy: Assessment, Treatment and Rehabilitation of Animals. UK: Blackwell Publishing; 2016. pp. 73-84

[60] O'Callaghan K. Lameness and associated pain in cattle—challenging traditional perceptions. In Practice. 2002;**24**(4):212

[61] Weishaupt MA. Adaptation strategies of horses with lameness. Veterinary Clinics of North America: Equine Practice. 2008;**24**(1):79-100

[62] Bicalho RC, Oikonomou G. Control and prevention of foot lameness associated with claw lesions in dairy cows. Livestock Science. 2013;**156**:96-105

[63] Green LE, Hedges VJ, Schukken YH, Blowey RW, Packington AJ. The impact of clinical lameness on the milk yield of dairy cows. Journal of Dairy Science. 2002;**85**(9):2250-2256

[64] Mulling CK, Green LE, Barker Z, Scaife J, Amory J, Speijers M, editors. Risk Factors Associated with Foot Foot Lameness in Dairy Cattle and a Suggested Approach for Foot Lameness Reduction. World Buiatrics Congress; 2006

[65] Broster C, Burn C, Barr A, Whay H. The range and prevalence of pathological abnormalities associated with foot lameness in working horses from developing countries. Equine Veterinary Journal. 2009;**41**:474-481

[66] Wiggers N, Nauwelaerts SLP, Hobbs SJ, Bool S, Wolschrijn CF, Back W. Functional locomotor consequences of uneven forefeet for trot symmetry in individual riding horses. PLoS One. 2015;**10**(2):e0114836

[67] Winter A. Foot lameness in sheep. Small Ruminant Research. 2008;**76**:149-153

[68] Ross MW, Dyson SJ. Diagnosis and management of foot lameness in the horse. Health Sciences. 2010;**36**:549-554

[69] Murray RC, Walters JM, Snart H, Dyson SJ, Parkin TDH. Identification of risk factors for lameness in dressage horses. Veterinary Journal. 2010;**184**(1):27-36

[70] Christodoulopoulos G. Foot lameness in dairy goats. Research in Veterinary Science. 2009;**86**(2):281-284

[71] Vermunt JJ. Subclinical laminitis in dairy-cattle. New Zealand Veterinary Journal. 1992;**40**(4):133-138

[72] Seitzinger AH, Traub-Dargatz J, Kane A, Kopral C, Morley P, Garber L, et al. A comparison of the economic costs of equine foot lameness, colic, and equine protozoal myeloencephalitis (EPM). In: Proceedings of the 9th International Symposium on Veterinary Epidemiology and Economics. 2000:1048-1050. https://naldc.nal.usda.gov/download/45446/PDF

[73] Moorman VJ, Reiser RF II, Peterson ML, McIlwraith CW, Kawcak CE. Effect of forelimb foot lameness on hoof kinematics of horses at a walk. American Journal of Veterinary Research. 2013;**74**:1192-1197

[74] Uprichard K, Boden L, Marshall J. An online survey to characterise spending patterns of horse owners and to quantify. Equine Veterinary Journal. 2014;**46**:4

[75] Cross B. New Survey Reveals UK's Current Equine Healthcare Problems. 2011. Available from: http://www.bluecross.org.uk/2000-84227/new-survey-reveals-uks-current-equine-healthcare-problems-.html

[76] Ireland JL, Clegg PD, McGowan CM, McKane SA, Chandler KJ, Pinchbeck GL. Disease prevalence in geriatric horses in the United Kingdom: Veterinary clinical assessment of 200 cases. Equine Veterinary Journal. 2012;**44**(1):101-106

[77] Wagner BA, Venkataraman S, Buettner GR. The rate of oxygen utilization by cells. Free Radical Biology & Medicine. 2011;**51**(3):700-712

[78] Kovac M, Litvin Y, Aliev R, Zakirova E, Rutland C, Kiyasov A, et al. Gene therapy using plasmid DNA encoding VEGF164 and FGF2 genes: A novel treatment of naturally occurring tendinitis and desmitis in horses. Frontiers in Pharmacology. 2018;**9**:978

[79] Weishaupt MA, Wiestner T, Hogg HP, Jordan P, Auer JA. Compensatory load redistribution of horses with induced weightbearing hindlimb lameness trotting on a treadmill. Equine Veterinary Journal. 2004;**36**(8):727-733

[80] Uhlir C, Lica T, Kubber P, Peham C, Scheidl M, Girtler D. Compensatory movements of horses with a stance phase foot lameness. Equine Veterinary Journal. 1997;**29**:102-105

[81] Keegan KG, Dent EV, Wilson DA, Janicek J, Kramer J, Lacarrubba A, et al. Repeatability of subjective evaluation of lameness in horses. Equine Veterinary Journal. 2010;**42**(2):92-97

[82] Malikides N, McGowan T, Pead M. Equine and canine foot lameness. In: McGowan C, Goff L, Stubbs N, editors. Animal Physiotherapy: Assessment, Treatment and Rehabilitation of Animals. UK: Wiley-Blackwell; 2007. pp. 73-101

[83] French KR, Pollitt CC. Equine laminitis: Congenital, hemidesmosomal plectin deficiency in a quarter horse foal. Equine Veterinary Journal. 2004;**36**(3):299-303

[84] Kummer M, Geyer H, Imboden I, Auer J, Lischer C. The effect of hoof trimming on radiographic measurements of the front feet of normal Warmblood horses. Veterinary Journal. 2006;**172**(1):58-66

[85] Holroyd K, Dixon JJ, Mair T, Bolas N, Bolt DM, David F, et al. Variation in foot conformation in lame horses with different foot lesions. Veterinary Journal. 2013;**195**(3):361-365

[86] Ryan T. Dorsal hoof wall grooving for the treatment of acute laminitis. Journal of Equine Veterinary Science. 2013;**33**:877

[87] Drumond B, Ginelli AMG, Faleiros RR, de Magalhaes JF, Coelhos CS. Hoof capsule distortion and radiographic measurements of the front feet in Mangalarga Marchador horses subjected to athletic training. Pferdeheilkunde. 2016;**32**(2):110-118

[88] Mungall BA, Pollitt CC. Zymographic analysis of equine laminitis. Histochemistry and Cell Biology. 1999;**112**(6):467-472

[89] Pollitt CC. Dysregulation of the lamellar basal epithelial cell in laminitis: Role of the cytoskeleton and cell junctions. In: Equine Laminitis. UK: Wiley Blackwell. Vol. 43. 2016. pp. 167-172

[90] Daradka M, Pollitt CC. Epidermal cell proliferation in the equine hoof

wall. Equine Veterinary Journal. 2004;**36**(3):236-241

[91] O'Grady SE, Castelijns HH. Sheared heels and the correlation to spontaneous quarter cracks. Equine Veterinary Education. 2011;**23**(5):262-269

[92] O'Grady SE. Farriery for the hoof with a sheared heel. Veterinary Clinics of North America: Equine Practice. 2012;**28**(2):381-392

[93] Holroyd K, Dixon JJ, Mair T, Bolas N, Weller R. Is there a relationship between foot conformation and foot lesions in lame horses? Journal of Equine Veterinary Science. 2013;**33**:858-859

[94] Newsome R, Green MJ, Bell NJ, Chagunda MGG, Mason CS, Rutland CS, et al. Linking bone development on the caudal aspect of the distal phalanx with lameness during life. Journal of Dairy Science. 2016;**99**(6):4512-4525

[95] Lean NE, Perkins NR, Ahern BJ. Comparison of conventional radiography and computed tomography as aids in the diagnosis of osteomyelitis in 11 foals. Australian Veterinary Journal. 2018;**96**(7):257-261

[96] Barrett MF, Selberg KT, Johnson SA, Hersman J, Frisbie DD. High field magnetic resonance imaging contributes to diagnosis of equine distal tarsus and proximal metatarsus lesions: 103 horses. Veterinary Radiology & Ultrasound. 2018;**59**(5):587-596

[97] Barrett MF, Manchon PT, Hersman J, Kawcak CE. Magnetic resonance imaging findings of the proximal metacarpus in quarter horses used for cutting: Retrospective analysis of 32 horses 2009-2012. Equine Veterinary Journal. 2018;**50**(2):172-178

[98] Kovac M, Litvin YA, Aliev RO, Zakirova EY, Rutland CS, Kiyasov AP, et al. Gene therapy using plasmid DNA encoding vascular endothelial growth factor 164 and fibroblast growth factor 2 genes for the treatment of horse tendinitis and desmitis: Case reports. Frontiers in Veterinary Science. 2017;**4**:168

[99] Keane M, Paul E, Sturrock C, Rauch C, Rutland C. Computed tomography in veterinary medicine: Currently published and tomorrow's vision. In: Halefoglu A, editor. Computed Tomography—Advanced Applications. Rijeka, Croatia: InTechOpen; 2017

[100] ICoVGAN (I.C.V.G.A.N). Nomina Anatomica Veterinaria. 6th revised edn. 2017. Available from: http://www.wava-amav.org/ [Accessed: December 5, 2017]

Chapter 3

Macroscopic, Radiographic and Histopathologic Changes of Claws with Laminitis and Laminitis-Related Disorders in Zero-Grazed Dairy Cows

James Nguhiu-Mwangi and Peter M.F. Mbithi

Abstract

Laminitis and laminitis-related claw disorders are prevalent in zero-grazed dairy cows. Confinement and limited movement influences claw size and shape. Abnormal claw size and shape causes imbalanced body weight distribution on the claws. Claw horn growth and wear is impaired, further aggravating laminitis disorders. The objective of this study was to determine: macroscopic disorders on the claws, as well as radiographic features and histopathologic changes on the claws with laminitis/laminitis-related disorders. A total of 159 dairy cow forelimb and hind limb feet (318 claws) were collected from an abattoir and a slaughter slab around Nairobi, Kenya. The claws were examined for macroscopic abnormalities, dorso-palmar or dorso-plantar radiography done, sagittal claw sections done, corium gross changes observed and corium tissues harvested for histopathology. Macroscopic disorders observed were: sole bruising, claw deformities, heel erosion, subclinical laminitis sole haemorrhages, double soles, chronic laminitis and white line separation. Radiographic changes observed mainly on distal phalanges were dilated vascular channels, irregular margins, exostoses/periostitis, distal phalangeal narrowing and lysis. Histopathologic changes in the corium included arterio-venous shunts, vascular wall rupture and thickening, vascular proliferation and thrombosis, corium and connective tissue oedema, degeneration, haemorrhages and spongiosis. Hence macroscopic, radiographic and histopathologic changes in laminitis claws affect locomotion.

Keywords: laminitis, sole bruising, corium, claw horn, vascular channels, pedal bone

1. Introduction

This chapter is about a descriptive presentation of the anatomic and physiological changes of the claws, which are the most vital part of the locomotor system of a dairy cow. The health of the claws allows free movement of the cow, which enhances adequate feeding time that leads to optimal reproduction and production, thus fulfilling the farmers' main purpose for keeping dairy cows. Over 80% of the dairy cattle herd in Kenya is under smallholder production [1], in most of which the dairy cows are kept in zero-grazing units with the animals confined for a long time [2]. Many of these smallholder zero-grazing units have improperly designed cattle-rearing structures, defective and unsuitable treading floors, inadequate and inconsistent nutritional diets, as well as generally poor husbandry and management practices [2]. All these factors interact synergistically and predispose dairy cows to laminitis and related non-infectious claw disorders [2–3]. It has been observed that housing of dairy cows in confinement leads to an increased prevalence of claw disorders. This is particularly true when the cows are confined on hard unyielding floors such as concrete, which exert immense pressure against the claws after loading them heavily under the opposing animal weight to ground forces [4–5]. Some of the non-infectious claw disorders such as white line separation, sole ulcer, double (underrun) soles, sole bruising/sole erosion and heel erosion can be the result or the cause of laminitis [6].

Laminitis tends to affect all the claws simultaneously in a single cow and when it advances to the chronic phase, there are obvious macroscopic claw deformities that make it difficult to reshape them to their normal anatomical appearance. These macroscopic deformities are often accompanied by irreversible damage to the internal structure of the claws [6–9]. Initially, laminitis occurs in a subtle clinically unrecognised state referred to as subclinical laminitis, which can only be discerned through claw trimming as sole and white line haemorrhages [6, 10, 11]. The haemorrhages are associated with pododermal microvasculature changes that lead to extravasation of serum and blood elements with subsequent staining of the internal layers of the horn next to the corium of the claw and later following horn-growth towards the surface of the sole, becomes visible externally as sole haemorrhages [6, 11, 12]. If claw trimming or keen observation is not done routinely in individual dairy cows, subclinical laminitis advances to chronic phase of laminitis and predisposes to laminitis-related non-infectious claw disorders with likelihood of occurrence of irreversible internal damage in the claws [6, 13].

The structural changes in the claws that result from laminitis and laminitis-related disorders are initially evident histologically, later they can be seen macroscopically and radiographically. Publications on comprehensive description of macroscopic, radiographic and histopathologic changes occurring in the claws during laminitis and laminitis-related disorders in dairy cows are scarce. The available publications describe scantly and separately the changes discernible through these three observational methods. The aim of this chapter is to comprehensively describe in a single publication the macroscopic, radiographic and histopathologic changes in the claws of dairy cows following subclinical and chronic laminitis, as well as laminitis-predisposed claw disorders. The study observed claws collected from abattoirs, which originated from slaughtered culled dairy cows. The publication also presents a comprehensive literature review on the structural changes affecting the claws from the various non-infectious disorders, especially laminitis.

2. Literature review

Laminitis is an aseptic diffuse inflammation of the pododerm (corium), which is the dermis of the claw. There is a progressive damage of the microvasculature of the corium, which compromises oxygen and nutrient supply to the corium cells, thus resulting in the production of low quality weak claw-horn [6, 14]. The low quality horn predisposes the claws of dairy cows to occurrence of various claw disorders associated with disruption of the claw-horn. These include sole ulcer, white line separation, double (underrun) soles, sole bruising (erosion) and heel erosion [6–8]. Claw-horn disruption is mainly thought to emanate from laminitis; hence, conclusion of association between laminitis and the claw disorders mentioned above [15]. Another factor that has the likelihood of causing claw-horn disruption in dairy cows is exertion of excessive forces on the germinal epithelium responsible for production of new claw horn. These excessive forces penetrate into the claw after depletion of adipose tissue in the digital cushion and the sole soft tissue thickness. The overall digital cushion and the sole soft tissue thickness become thinner to the extent that they cannot dissipate the concussion forces [16]. These authors have stated that the likelihood of having claw lesions has been associated with thin digital cushion. Impaired claw function has also been traced to weakened claw structures including subcutaneous tissue (digital cushion), dermis (corium) and suspensory apparatus. These lead to the damage of the vascular system of the dermis, disruption of dermal-epidermal junction as well as the horn producing cells [17].

The prevailing factors during the peri-parturient period predispose dairy cows to likelihood of more claw-horn wear and negative horn-growth. This effect leads to thinned soles that subsequently allow pressure penetration into the corium exacerbating its fragility and injury, consequently producing poor quality horn. Other structural changes in the claws occurring during the peri-parturient period in dairy cows include the slight shifting of the distal phalanx within the claw horn capsule. The distal phalanx rotates and sinks lower into the claw capsule. This movement of the distal phalanx is incriminated on the rising levels of the enzyme "hoofase" that occurs in the peri-parturient period, which causes more flexibility of the connective tissue suspending this bone within the claw horn capsule [18]. Studies have shown that sole haemorrhages were absent in heifers that had not calved, while these haemorrhages occurred after the heifers calved [19]. This confirms the role played by peri-parturient factors in predisposing to the occurrence claw-horn lesions. During the peri-parturient period, digital cushion and sole soft tissue become thinner, hence the germinal epithelium of the corium becomes predisposed to pressure. This results in production of poor quality horn as well as reduced horn production, especially the horn of the sole [16]. The alterations of thickness of sole soft tissue during the peri-parturient period are thought to be influenced by reproductive hormones relaxin and oestrogens. These hormones cause activation of the enzymes metalloproteinases, which degrade collagen [20]. The scores of lesions in the sole are higher during the postpartum period. These lesions decrease in the late lactation. Wider outward angle of the hind limbs caused by the size and weight of the udder in early lactation, predisposes the claws especially the lateral claws to occurrence of lesions [21]. Apart from hormonal factors during early postpartum period and in early lactation, metabolic changes associated with parturition and lactation similarly contributes to increased locomotion as well as lesion scores in dairy cows [20]. Lesions causing structural changes in the claws are more common and with higher locomotion scores in dairy cows that have had greater number of parities/lactations, especially five or more lactations [21].

Dairy cow housing-related factors are major contributors to the occurrence of claw lesions and structural changes. This is particularly common in the more confined dairy cows such as the smallholder zero-grazing units [2]. The type of floor on which the cows live and walk is the main housing factor predisposing them to develop claw lesions. This is determined by either rough or slippery floor texture [22], as well as defective concrete floors with small or large pot-holes [2]. The distribution of the weight of the cow on the claws is influenced by the hardness of the floor. Hard floors cause most of the animal weight to be loaded on the abaxial wall of the claws, while soft yielding floors lead to significant distribution of weight to the sole. The overall effect of the weight force against the mechanical pressure from the floor depends on the architectural arrangement of the claw wall determined by the interrelationship arrangement of tubular, intertubular and laminar horn cells. The numerical density of the horn tubules determines the differences in the stiffness and elasticity of the various parts of the claw horn capsule. The degree of the effect of the mechanical forces from the animal weight and floor pressure is associated with the degree of horn capsule elasticity and stiffness [22]. The longer the dairy cow stands on hard unyielding floor such as concrete, the more the likelihood of developing claw lesions [23]. Besides the pressure transmitted to the inside of the claws from the hard floors, the floor abrasiveness has a significant contribution to the occurrence of claw lesions, mainly due to excessive wearing of the claw-horn [24]. The claws are particularly prone to this abrasiveness of the floor when the horn produced is weak following bouts of laminitis [8]. Conversely, the claw-horn does not wear off when the cow lives and walks on soft yielding floors such as earthen floors or straw yards. This leads to inevitable overgrowth of the claws with subsequent overloading of the region towards the heel bulb, which is soft, hence the ease of transmission of pressure to the inner claw tissues, thus damaging them. The result of this is the production of poor quality horn [23]. All these factors have an overall effect of causing changes in the claw shape as well as structural changes internally.

3. Materials and methods

3.1 The study area

The study was carried out in the peri-urban areas of Nairobi City in the Republic of Kenya. The area was chose owing to its high number of smallholder zero-grazing dairy units. The high number of smallholder zero-grazing dairy units is instigated by the availability of market to which farmers sell milk and the value-added dairy products. The market is from the high number of city dwellers and workers. Nairobi and its peri-urban region have an area of 696 km^2 with estimated over 2.5 million people. It is located between latitude 01° 18′S and longitude 36° 45′E with an altitude of 1798 m above sea level. The estimated annual rainfall is maximum of 765 mm in the season from March to June, and a minimum of 36 mm in the season from October to December. The other areas from where samples for the study were collected included an abattoir in Kiserian centre of Kajiado County, Kenya and a slaughter slab in Wangige area of Kiambu County, Kenya.

3.2 The study design

This was a prospective abattoir study in which claws were collected from slaughtered dairy cows. Claws from an abattoir and a slaughter slab were subject to the number of dairy cows slaughtered per given time.

3.3 The sample size and sample selection

The two places selected from which dairy cow claws were collected included Kiserian abattoir and wangige slaughter slab. They were purposively selected based on the findings of an earlier pilot survey indicating that culled dairy cows were regularly slaughtered in these two places. Slaughter of dairy cows is not commonly done, hence the difficulties in getting their claws. The dairy cows send to slaughter were culled as a result of reasons related with poor production, poor reproductive performance, non-treatable problems and old age. The combined number of dairy cow feet collected from both slaughter places was 159, which made a total of 318 claws. A total of 96 feet were from Wangige slaughter slab, which had more dairy cows slaughtered and 63 were from Kiserian abattoir. Among the 159 feet, 109 were from the hind limbs and 50 from the forelimbs. More hind limb claws were collected based on the literature knowledge that they suffer more problems than forelimb claws. Since only a small number of dairy cows are slaughtered, it necessitated collection of the available claws without any random selection. History indicated that all the cows from which the claws were collected had been kept under zero-grazing system.

3.4 Examination of the claws for data collection

Each of claws collected from the abattoir and the slaughter slab was thoroughly washed. Observation of gross appearing lesions was done. Each lesion/abnormality was recorded in data collection sheets. Each claw was radiographed in dorso-palmar or dorso-plantar views. The radiographs were viewed and examined thoroughly. All radiographic changes seen were recorded. Owing to the time lapse between slaughter and examination, the claws were partially desiccated by loss of their water content, making trimming difficult. Therefore, after radiography, the area covered by the horn capsule was dipped in water for 2–3 h to make them softer for facilitation of trimming. Trimming was done by removing 2–3 mm of the horn of the sole, while observation of any lesion on the sole was made. All lesions were recorded. About 10 claws with subclinical laminitis and another 10 claws with chronic laminitis were purposively selected. Sagittal sections of all these 20 selected claws were done starting from the fetlock joint level through proximal, middle and distal phalanges. All gross lesions observed in the exposed corium and the phalanges after sagittal section were recorded.

The horn of the sole was removed from each claw using a knife to expose the corium of the sole fully. Sections of about 5 mm thickness of the corium specimens were harvested in transverse and longitudinal planes from each of the claw samples. The corium specimens were further sectioned into 1–2 millimetre pieces, which were dehydrated using ascending concentrations of absolute isopropyl alcohol, that started from 80 to 100%. Clearing of the tissues was done in xylene, then embedded in paraffin wax, blocked on wooden chunks, followed by fixing on the microtome. The tissues that were in paraffin wax blocks were cut into 5 μm thick pieces. From each block, four pieces of 5 μm thick tissues were made. This was followed by dewaxing the tissue sections in xylene and hydrated using graded alcohol whose concentration was from 100 to 50%. It was cleared in xylene, alcohol and washed in water. The tissues were stained with haematoxylin and eosin (H&E). Following dehydration, they were mounted on microscope slides and cover slips with Destrene 80, dibutyl phthalate and Xylene (DPX) mountant according to Ref. [25]. The slides were examined under light microscope using ×10, ×40 and ×100 objective lenses. The results were recorded and photomicrographs taken as necessary. The control in this study was done by comparing the findings in the normal claws with those that had lesions or were abnormal. The corium samples from claws that did not show signs of subclinical or chronic laminitis were processed using similar procedure as the test specimens and used as controls.

3.5 Data management and analysis

Claw lesions were given numerical codes for ease of entry into the computer. The prevalence of claw lesions was computed using Microsoft Office Excel data analysis tool as the number of dairy cow abattoir feet/claws showing a specific type of lesion divided by the total number of feet/claws examined multiplied by 100 to make it into percentage. Percentages of occurrence of radiographic changes were calculated by dividing the number of claws showing a specific radiographic feature by the total number of claws examined through radiography multiplied by 100. The percentages of histopathologic changes were calculated out of the number of claws with subclinical laminitis and chronic laminitis selected for histological evaluation.

3.6 Ethical approval

Permission to collect claws from the abattoir and the slaughter slab was granted by the Director of Veterinary Services, Kenya through the Veterinary Officers in the two places, respectively. The ethical approval of the proposal was given by the Biosafety, Animal Use and Ethics Committee of the Faculty of Veterinary Medicine, University of Nairobi, Kenya.

4. Results of the study

4.1 Macroscopic changes

Various macroscopic lesions/disorders were observed in the claws collected from the abattoir and from the slaughter slab. These included claw deformities (consisting of overgrown claws, flattened claws, concave dorsal wall and corkscrew claws) at a prevalence of 78.0% (n = 248) of the claws. Sole bruising (erosion) was seen in 44.0% (n = 140) of the claws and heel erosion at 41.5% (n = 132) of the claws. Others included subclinical laminitis (only evidenced by localised sole haemorrhages after a thin layer of the sole was trimmed-off), which was found in 34.6% (n = 110) of the claws, double (underrun) soles in 23.2% (n = 74) and chronic laminitis (evidenced by some types of claw deformities and more diffuse severe sole haemorrhages) in 21.4 (n = 68) of the claws. The rest of the lesions with low prevalence can be seen in **Table 1**.

Severe congestion of the sole corium was observed in the claws that had subclinical laminitis as well as those that had chronic laminitis. The congestion was more severe in the claws that had chronic laminitis than in those that had subclinical laminitis. On sagittal section, the pedal bone appeared dark red in claws with laminitis when compared to the normal claws.

Sole bruising (erosion) caused severe thinning of the horn of the sole, which made the corium to be positioned extremely close to the surface of the sole. This was clearly evident after the sagittal section in comparison to the normal claw (**Figure 1**). The thinning of the horn was more evident in sole bruising than in heel bruising (erosion). The claws that had sole bruising were also found to manifest sole haemorrhages. When the necrotic appearing horn of the bruised sole was trimmed, the protective function of the remaining horn was compromised due to the degree of thinness. Double soles and the degree of sole erosion became clearer after claw trimming was done (**Figure 2**).

Claw deformities ranged from mild to severe and usual deformities that clearly impaired the normal gait causing the cows to show obvious signs of lameness. Depending on the extent and degree of deformity, weight distribution on the claws was grossly unequal and not according to the natural normalcy.

Claw lesions/disorders	Number of cow feet (n = 159)	Number of claws (n = 318)	Prevalence (%)
Sole bruising	124	248	78.0
Claw deformities	70	140	44.0
Heel erosion	66	132	41.5
Subclinical laminitis	55	110	34.6
Double (underrun) sole	37	74	23.3
Chronic laminitis	34	68	21.4
White line separation	26	52	16.4
Foreign bodies	5	10	3.1
Sole ulcer	1	2	0.6
Claw infection	1	2	0.6

Table 1.
Percentage occurrence of macroscopic lesions/disorders out of 159 dairy cow feets (318 claws) collected from Kiserian abattoir and Wangige Slaughter slab in Kajiado County and Kiambu County, Kenya, respectively.

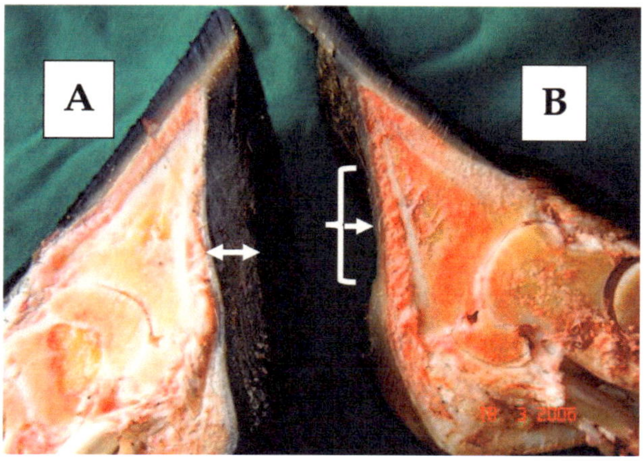

Figure 1.
Sagittal section of a normal claw (A) showing adequate thickness of the horn of the sole (double-headed arrow); and a claw with severe sole bruising (erosion) (B) showing extremely thinned horn of the sole with the corium very close to the treading surface (brace and arrow).

4.2 Radiographic features

The claws that were collected from the abattoir and the slaughter slab had varying prevalence of radiographic changes that occurred in the distal phalanges, particularly in those that had chronic laminitis. Other radiographic changes seen affected the blood vessels. Out of the 159 abattoir feet samples examined, 25.8% (n = 41) had more than one radiographic lesion. The most prevalent and consistently seen radiographic features were: prominently dilated vascular channels in 60.8% (n = 97), prominent but not dilated vascular channels in 24.1% (n = 38), irregular pedal bone margins in 13.9% (n = 22), pedal bone exostoses in 9.4% (n = 15) and narrowed/tapering pedal bone in 5.7% (n = 9) of the 159 dairy cow feet samples. Other radiographic features seen occurred in less than 5% (**Table 2**). Radiographic changes in

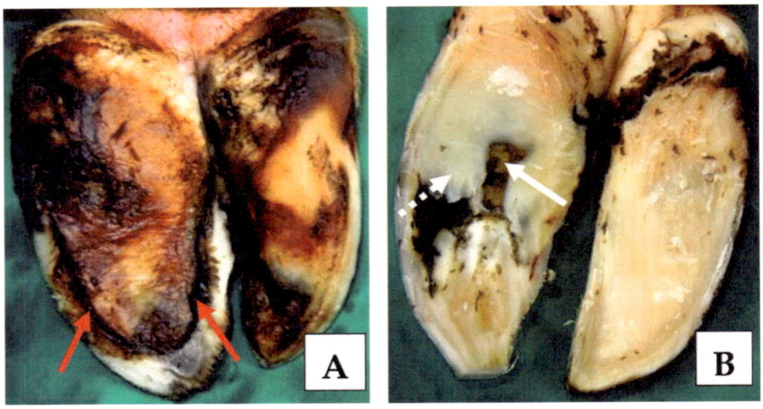

Figure 2.
Claw with double (underrun) soles whose margins are clearly distinct as shown (bold arrows) in A. The thin inner sole in B is exposed (bold arrow) after trimming-off part of the outer superficial sole (dotted arrow). This occurred concurrently with chronic laminitis in some dairy cow claws.

laminitis and other claw disorders were only observed in the distal phalanx. The middle and proximal phalanges did not show any changes. Vascular channels were markedly prominent in the distal ends of pedal bones of the claws that had laminitis.

These were more prominently dilated in claws with chronic laminitis, visible in claws with subclinical laminitis and hardly visible in claws without laminitis (**Figure 3**). The margins of the pedal bone from claws with chronic laminitis were small irregular serrations towards the distal end of the bone. The pedal bones from claws with subclinical laminitis and other laminitis-related disorders did not show any irregular margins (**Figure 4**).

Slight osseous overgrowths were seen on the periosteum at the distal parts of distal phalanges in some of the claws with chronic laminitis. Similar findings were seen in some of the claws with severe deformities. This radiographic feature seemed like exostosis (**Figure 5**). One of the claws with chronic laminitis had pedal bone with exostosis on the plantar surface (**Figure 5**). None of the claws with subclinical laminitis and other laminitis-related lesions had bone periosteal overgrowths.

Radiographic lesion	Number of feet samples (n = 159)	Number of claws (n = 318)	Percentage occurrence (%)
Dilated vascular channels	96	192	60.4
Prominent but not dilated vascular channels	38	76	23.9
Irregular pedal bone margins	22	44	13.8
Exostoses of pedal bone	15	30	9.4
Narrowed (tapering) pedal bone	9	18	5.7
Absent pedal bone apex	4	8	2.5
Fractured pedal bone	3	6	1.9
Periostitis of pedal bone	2	4	1.3
Osteolysis of pedal bone	1	2	0.6

The changes were observed in claws with laminitis and/or laminitis-related lesions/disorders.

Table 2.
Radiographic changes observed out of the 159 dairy cow feet examined from Kiserian abattoir, Kajiado County and Wangige slaughter slab, Kiambu County, Kenya.

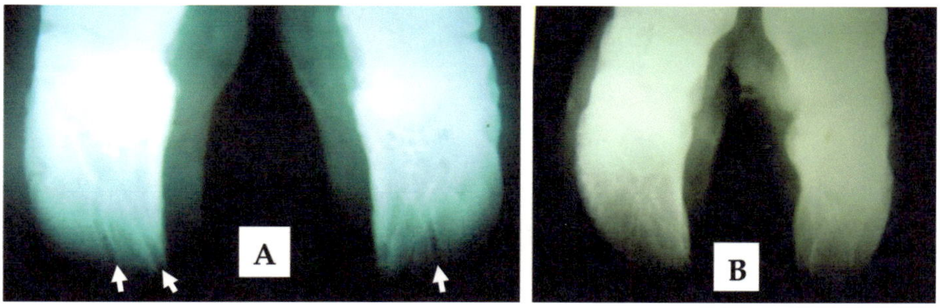

Figure 3.
Prominently dilated vascular channels (arrows) seen in claws with chronic laminitis (A), compared with unnoticeable vascular channels in a normal non-laminitis claw (B).

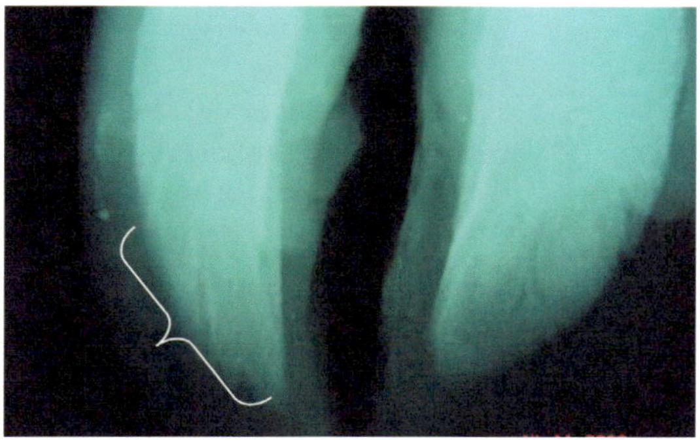

Figure 4.
Irregular serrations of the distal margin of the pedal bone (area with brace enclosure) in some of the claws that had chronic laminitis. Compare with the ipsilateral claw, which shows no serrations on the distal margin.

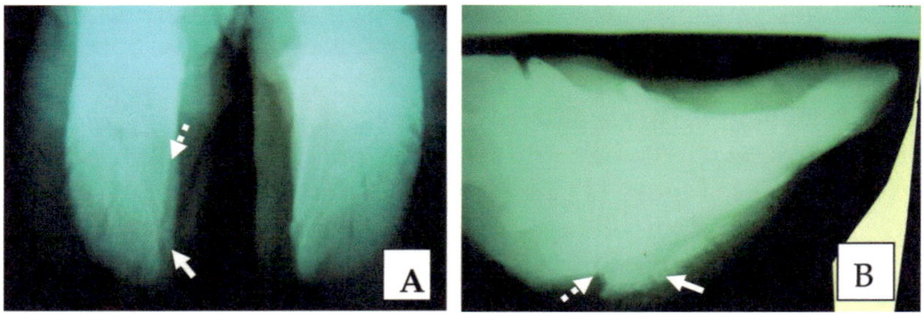

Figure 5.
Periosteal-like exostosis (bold arrow) with definite margin (dotted arrow) on the medial side of pedal bone in A. Exostosis (bold arrow) on the plantar surface of pedal bone with definite margin (dotted arrow) in B. These exostoses were found in some of the pedal bones from claws of dairy cows with laminitis.

Extreme tapering of the distal parts of the pedal bone was observed in some of the claws that had chronic laminitis with severe deformities such as twisted toe. The pedal bone was markedly narrowed (**Figure 6**). The other laminitis-related disorders including subclinical laminitis did not show this radiographic feature.

Another radiographic feature seen in claws with chronic laminitis and extreme twisting of the toe is absence of the sharp apex of the distal phalanx. The apex of the bone appeared more rounded than the normal ipsilateral claw (**Figure 7**). Claws with chronic laminitis but without deformity of the toe did not have this pedal apical feature. One of the radiographic features observed in claws with excessive sole bruising and heel erosion coupled with claw deformities was fracture-like fissures of the distal

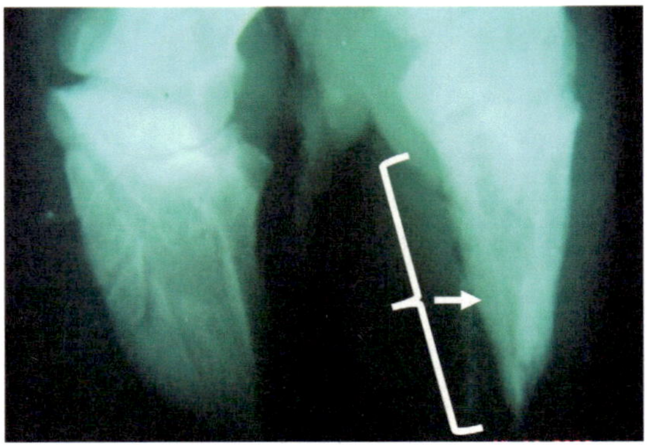

Figure 6.
Narrowed pedal bone (arrow) whose extent of tapering is shown (brace). The pedal bone of the ipsilateral claw is normal width. This radiographic change was observed in dairy cow claws with laminitis.

phalanx. The fissure was small and the part that appeared like bone fragment was still aligned to the entire bone (**Figure 8**). One distal phalanx was found to have osteolysis, which was clearly manifested by radiolucency of the bone appearing like the bone has a large medullary cavity (**Figure 9**), which is naturally absent in the pedal bone.

4.3 Histopathological features

Arteriovenous shunts (AVs), disruption of the dermal-epidermal junction, rupture of the vascular wall, vascular thrombosis and vascular proliferation were the main histological changes frequently observed in the claws with laminitis and the laminitis-related lesions. Other histological changes observed but rare included oedema in the dermis of the sole, connective tissue oedema, thickened arterial wall, degeneration and necrosis of the connective tissue that supports the distal phalanx, damage of the epidermal cells, spongiosis of the stratum basale and stratum spinosum, corium haemorrhages, connective tissue degeneration and enlargement of veins (**Table 3**).

Arteriovenous shunts (**Figure 10**) were observed in 40 and 50% of the corium specimens from claws with subclinical laminitis and chronic laminitis, respectively. Vascular wall damage (**Figure 11**) and dermal-epidermal junction disruption (**Figure 12**) were each observed in 30 and 50% of the corium specimens from claws with subclinical and chronic laminitis, respectively. Spongiosis was seen in 30% of

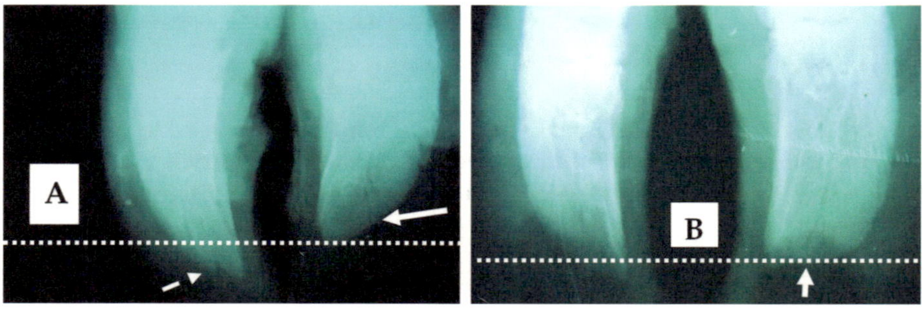

Figure 7.
A rounded (missing) apex of the pedal bone (bold arrow) making the bone look shorter than the ipsilateral pedal bone as shown (dotted line) in A and B. The projected apical part of the ipsilateral pedal bone is slightly irregular with serrations (dashed arrow). These radiographic changes were observed in dairy cow claws that had laminitis.

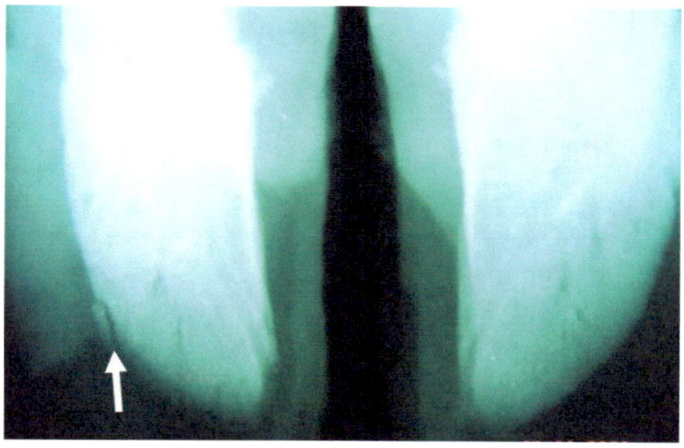

Figure 8.
A small fracture-like fissure (arrow) observed in three pedal bones from dairy cow claws that had laminitis.

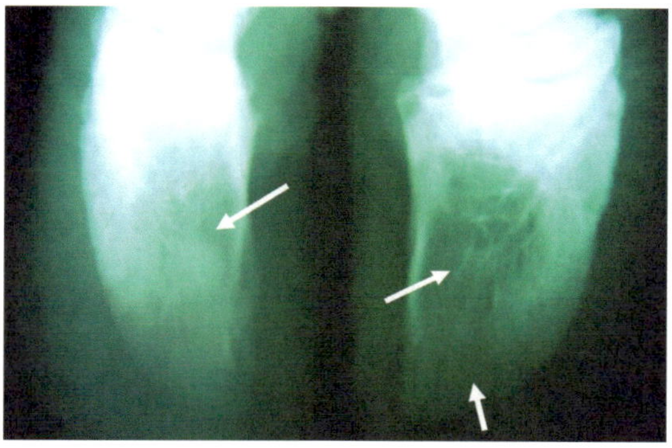

Figure 9.
Pedal bones showing radiolucent areas representing bone lysis (arrows). The areas look similar to medullary cavity, which is normally absent in normal pedal bones. This was observed in one dairy cow claw that had chronic laminitis.

Histopathological lesions	Prevalence (%) in subclinical laminitis (n = 10)	Prevalence (%) in chronic laminitis (n = 10)
Arteriovenous shunts	40	50
Vascular wall damage	30	50
Dermal-epidermal junction disruption	30	50
Vascular thrombosis	40	100
Vascular proliferation	30	30
Oedema of corium and connective tissue	20	20
Vascular wall thickness	30	10
Connective tissue degeneration	0	30
Corium haemorrhages	10	20
Spongiosis	0	30

The claws were collected from Kiserian abattoir of Kajiado County and Wangige slaughter slab of Kiambu County, Kenya.

Table 3.
Histopathological changes observed in the corium tissue specimens harvested from dairy cow claws with subclinical laminitis and chronic laminitis.

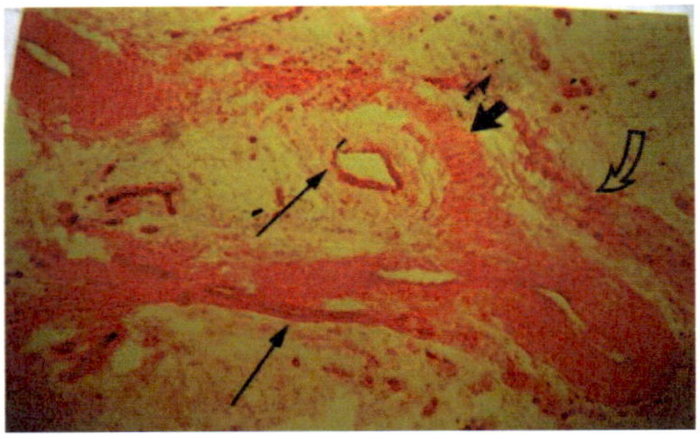

Figure 10.
Arteriovenous shunts shown by branching out of the wall of the artery (bold arrow) and inclusion of veins within the arterial wall boundaries (thin arrows) and the position of capillary-beds (curved arrows). These changes were seen in the corium of dairy cow claws with laminitis. (H&E stain, ×400).

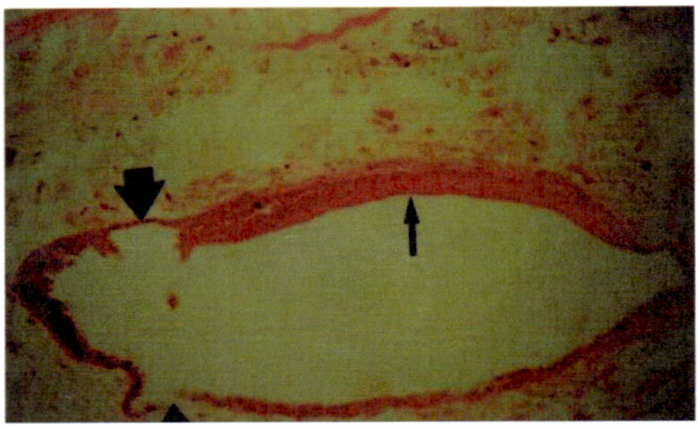

Figure 11.
A vein showing damaged wall (thick arrow) and a thrombus attached to the wall (thin arrow). This was a common feature in the corium of dairy cow claws with laminitis. (H&E stain, ×400).

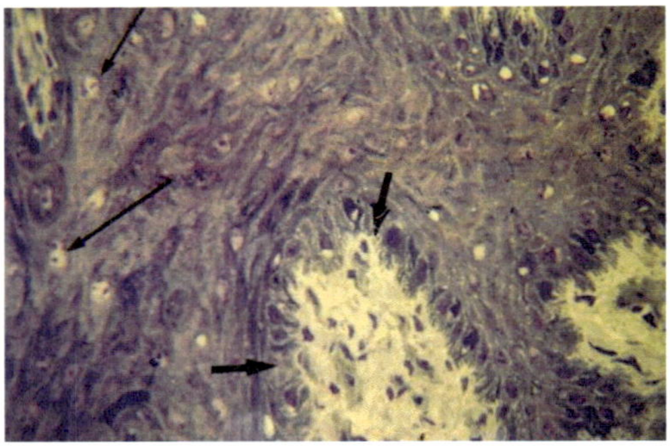

Figure 12.
Dermal-epidermal junction disruption shown by areas where the cells are not in contact and continuous with each other (short arrows). Intracellular oedema (spongiosis) (long thin arrows). These were common findings in cases of claws with laminitis. (Toluidine blue stain, ×400).

the specimens from claws with chronic laminitis (**Figure 12**), but it was not seen in claws with subclinical laminitis. Vascular wall damage was seen more regularly in the arterioles and venules than in the larger blood vessels. Endothelial disruption was seen more frequently than damage of the rest of the vascular wall. Rupture of the entire thickness of blood vessel wall followed by haemorrhage into the surrounding tissues was seen in 10 and 20% of the corium specimens from claws with subclinical and chronic laminitis, respectively. All the histological changes mentioned above were more common, extensive and severe in the corium specimens from claws with chronic laminitis than in those with subclinical laminitis.

Vascular thrombosis (**Figure 13**) was found in 70% of all corium specimens. All the corium specimens from claws with chronic laminitis were found to have vascular thrombosis, but only 40% of the corium specimens from claws with subclinical laminitis. Thickened vascular wall particularly of the arteries was found in 40% of the specimens, 30% from claws with subclinical laminitis (**Figure 13**). The vascular layer that appeared more prominently thickened was tunica media and in some of the specimens, it was evident that this thickening was due to oedema. Degeneration of the connective tissue that supports the distal phalanx was observed in 40% of the specimens, all of which were from claws with chronic laminitis. Oedema in the dermis of the sole and in the connective tissue (**Figure 14**) was found in 40% of the specimens, half from claws with subclinical laminitis and half from claws with chronic laminitis. Evidence of haemorrhages in the corium was found in 30 and 10% of the specimens from claws with chronic laminitis and subclinical laminitis, respectively. Mild degeneration of the sole connective tissue was seen in 30% of the specimens from claws with chronic laminitis (**Figure 15**). In 20% of all the specimens of claws with subclinical laminitis and chronic laminitis, the veins had enlargements that appeared like dilatations.

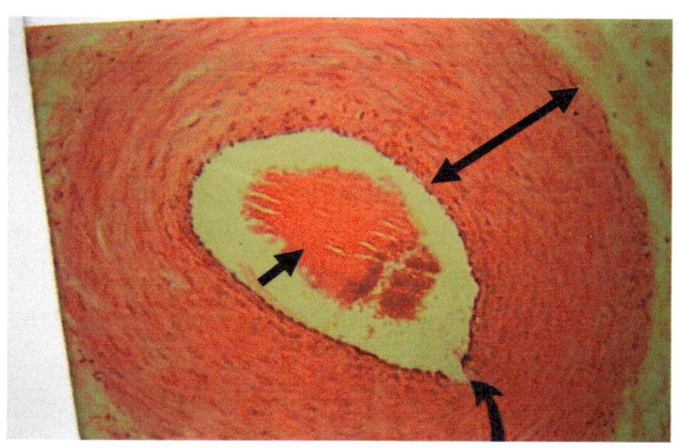

Figure 13.
Thickened arterial wall (double-headed arrow), disrupted arterial endothelium (curved arrow) and a thrombus in the lumen of the artery (single-headed arrow) (H&E stain, ×400). This was a feature observed in the corium vasculature of dairy cow claws with laminitis. (H&E stain, ×400).

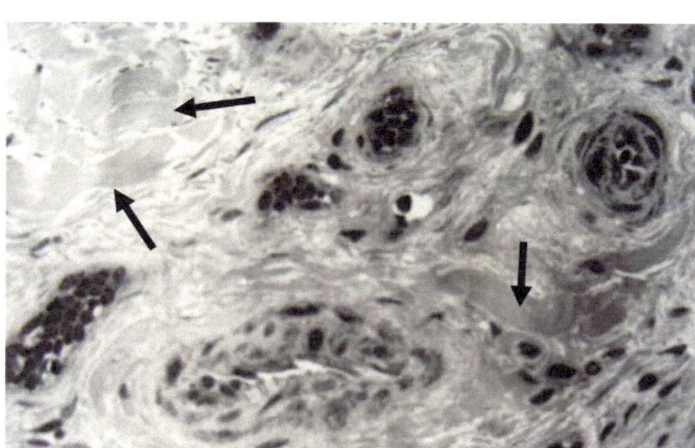

Figure 14.
Connective tissue oedema (arrows) seen in the corium of dairy cow claws with laminitis. (H&E stain, ×400).

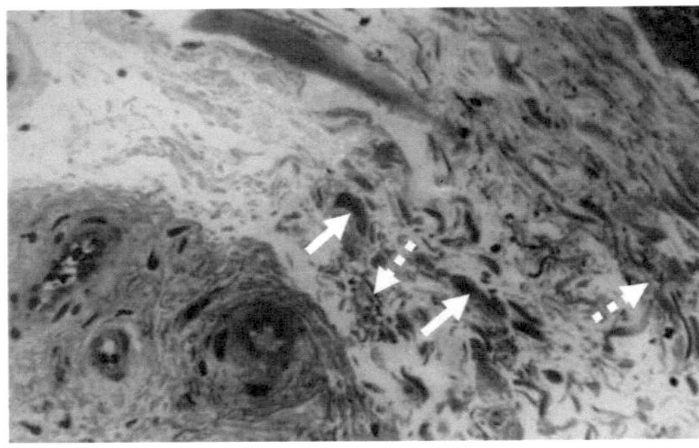

Figure 15.
Connective tissue degeneration manifested by deeply stained degenerated fibroblasts (bold arrows) and fibres (dotted arrows) in the histological sections of the corium of dairy cow claws with chronic laminitis (Toluidine blue stain, ×200).

5. Discussion

Laminitis influences the occurrence of other claw lesions and disorders such as sole ulcer, white line separation, double (underrun) soles, sole bruising (erosion) and heel erosion [6–8, 15, 26]. The occurrence of laminitis in dairy cows is predisposed by an interactive array of multiple risk factors [2, 6]. The high prevalence of laminitis and laminitis-related lesions/disorders in the dairy cow claws from Kiserian abattoir and Wangige slaughter slab can probably be attributed to the types of modern farming systems adopted in the dairy business enterprises in which the dairy cows are confined for long hours on hard unyielding concrete floors with much concentrate feeding. Such housing and feeding factors have been incriminated as risk factors for the development of laminitis [6, 7, 23, 27, 28]. The smallholder zero-grazing dairy units expose the cows to additional suboptimal management conditions such as prolonged presence of slurry, lack of claw trimming, and defective concrete floors apart from concentrate feeding [2, 8].

The high prevalence of prominently dilated vascular channels in the distal phalanges of the claws with laminitis particularly chronic laminitis corroborates previous documented observations that dilated vascular channels are consistent observations in subclinical and chronic laminitis. These previous reports indicated that in laminitis, both dilated and non-dilated vascular channels could be found [29]. The more prominent and excessively dilated vascular channels seen in chronic laminitis compared to subclinical laminitis could probably be associated with the greater damage internally in the claws during chronic laminitis [8].

The observed exostoses in the distal phalanges of claws with chronic laminitis are similar to an old report, which found exostosis in the pyramidal process of the pedal bone [30]. Occurrence of these exostoses could be associated with periostitis of the distal phalanges owing to prolonged inflammatory stimuli in chronic laminitis [8]. Although the factors associated with exostosis were not determined in this study, non-infective claw-horn disruption lesions (CHDL) have previously been incriminated as being associated with extra bone development particularly on the caudal aspect of the distal phalanx. The cows that had suffered chronic lameness from CHDL were found to have greater extra bone growth on the caudal aspect of distal phalanx, which was verified both by morphological gross observations and and histologically. This extra bone growth was more in quantity on the lateral claws of the hind limbs and medial claws of the forelimbs [31]. Extra bone development on the distal phalanges was reported to be positively correlated with the age of the cow [32]. Since, the claws in the current study were from culled aged dairy cows and had signs of non-infective claw-horn disorders, the findings corroborate these previous reports. It has also been suggested that infectious claw lesions are not associated with extra bone growth in the distal phalanges [31].

Narrowing (tapering) of the pedal bone towards the apex is a feature not previously described. Closely resembling this, is the atrophy of pedal bone reported in cattle with chronic laminitis [33]. This narrowing of the pedal bone could probably be attributed to osseous tissue necrosis (osteosis), which is linked to the deprivation of the nutrients and oxygen especially when local blood supply is compromised similar to what occurs in the claws with chronic laminitis [34]. Thromboembolic blockage of blood vessels with chronic local anaemia may also lead to osteosis unless supplemented by the presence of effective collateral circulation. However, bones have poor and inefficient collateral circulation owing to small anastomosing vasculature incapable of adequate compensatory dilatation. This makes them prone to osseous ischaemia that leads to necrosis with subsequent resorption of the necrotic bone by the osteoclasts [34]. If this process takes place during chronic laminitis with extreme twisting of the toe, then there would be likelihood of pedal bone narrowing. This could also explain the observation in some of the pedal bones that had absence of the apex from claws with chronic laminitis. Moreover, atrophy of the pedal bone reported previously in chronic laminitis could also be incriminated in the pedal apical absence [33].

Pedal bone osteolysis could be associated with reduced overall density of the bone in chronic laminitis as reported previously with crooked toe [30]. Productive periostitis of the pedal bone could be a response to irritation of the periosteum in claws with excessive inflammation of the corium in chronic laminitis. This could also lead to the irregular margins observed towards the distal margins of the pedal bone. The pedal bones in the lateral claws of the hind limbs had more severe and extensive radiographic changes than those of the medial claws. This corroborates earlier reports of higher prevalence and severity of lesions occurring on the lateral claws of the hind limbs of cattle than the medial claws [35, 36].

The observation of arteriovenous shunts (AVs) in this study was similar to previous reports in which the same was found [6, 37]. These shunts are normally not seen in healthy claws [38]. The arteriovenous shunts mainly involved the arterioles and venules. Arteriovenous shunts could be attributed to the fact that narrowed vessels have a likelihood of being affected by changes in blood pressure involved in the microcirculation of the corium [39], in which the arteriovenous shunts form as structural change adjustment [40].

The vascular damage in this study, which affected mainly dermal arteries, has been reported previously [38]. The pressure build-up from intermittent vasodilation and vasoconstriction of the corium microvasculature during laminitis may be the cause of this vascular damage [6]. The build-up of local blood pressure due to the initial increase in blood flow and pooling of blood within the corium capillary-bed, may lead to blood vessel rupture followed by haemorrhages and seepage of serum [6]. This eventually leads to the observation of haemorrhages seen macroscopically on the sole in cases of laminitis.

Thickening of vascular wall particularly of the arteries was similar to proliferated tunica intima, hypertrophied tunica media and fibrotic tunica adventitia reported earlier in laminitis [41]. The thickened arterial wall would obviously interfere with the function of the blood vessel. Vascular thrombosis is an almost invariable occurrence in the corium of claws with laminitis whether subclinical or chronic [6, 42]. The formation of thrombi might result from vascular damage particularly the endothelium, or from influence of the vasoactive substances within vascular circulation [6, 43]. Numerous capillary network is normal in the corium of the claws [40]. However, the vascular proliferation observed in this study, which led to an increased capillary network, could be a response to inflammatory reaction occurring in laminitis [14]. Enlarged veins seen only in chronic laminitis, which remained widely open appeared like venous dilatation rather than thickening of the wall. This feature has not been described previously in laminitis.

Oedema that was seen in the corium and in the connective tissue of the sole has been reported previously [6]. It occurs as a result of rising capillary pressure together with post-capillary resistance, which enhances transvascular fluid seepage followed by increased pressure within the tissues. Digital venous constrictions are thought to be the initial step in these processes [39]. Subsequently, oedema expands the corium, which causes pain that leads to lameness seen in laminitis [6, 44].

Although chronic degenerative change in the bovine corium of the claw has been reported in chronic laminitis previously [45], the disruptive connective tissue damage particularly involving fibroblasts has not been reported previously. This disruptive damage is probably a degenerative change associated with enzymatic action of matrix metalloproteinases (MMPs) and gelatinolytic protease known as hoofase [46]. It may also be a biochemical alteration in the connective tissue [20]. The degenerative disruption of the connective tissue was observed only in specimens from claws with chronic laminitis.

Disruption of the dermal-epidermal junction is an invariable finding in subclinical and chronic laminitis owing to compromised microvasculature of the corium, which causes nutrients and oxygen to be diminished to the extent of not reaching the epidermal cells. This causes breakdown of the stratum germinativum in the epidermis, the corium becomes degenerated and eventually a breakdown in dermal-epidermal junction that results in separation between the stratum germinativum and the corium [44]. Spongiosis and hyperplasia of the epidermis have not been reported previously. Both of these histological changes occurred in subclinical as well as in chronic laminitis. Probably, they are due to inflammation triggered by pressure irritation on the soft tissues located between the pedal bone and the horn of the sole after the claw comes into contact with the hard treading surface when the cow is in standing posture or in locomotion.

Previous studies have shown that laminitis and laminitis-related claw disorders have various cow-level and farm management-level risk factors [2, 6–8]. Although the cows whose claws were used in this study had been pregnant several times, the number of pregnancies and the stage of lactation were not ascertained from the zero-grazing units in which they were kept. It would therefore be recommended that further study be conducted relating macroscopic, radiographic and histopathologic findings on the claws with number of parities, state of pregnancy and stage of lactation of the cows. This will reveal the nature of correlation between these factors, thus indicating the factors exacerbating morphological changes on the dairy cow claws. This should also include correlation with the seasons of the year.

6. Conclusions

The study concluded that claw disorders are prevalent in dairy cows kept under zero-grazing system. The most commonly occurring macroscopic disorders are sole bruising (erosion), claw deformities, heel erosion, double soles, both subclinical and chronic laminitis and white line separation. The radiographic changes found in the claws were mainly associated with chronic laminitis. These occurred on the pedal bone and included dilated vascular channels, irregular bone margins, narrowing of the bone towards the apex and osteolysis. The histopathologic changes were common in the corium of both subclinical and chronic laminitis claws, which included mainly changes in the vasculature such as venular wall damage, arterial wall thickening, vascular thrombosis, connective tissue changes including oedema and degeneration. Most of these changes are evidently irreversible, hence making dairy cows suffering chronic laminitis coupled with extreme claw deformities to have poor prognoses.

Acknowledgements

We are grateful to the University of Nairobi Deans Committee for provision of funds to carry out this research. We thank the Chairman of the Department of Clinical Studies for allowing us the use of Departmental laboratory and imaging facilitation to carry out this research.

Conflict of interest

There is no conflict of interest for this project and publication whatsoever.

Author details

James Nguhiu-Mwangi[1*] and Peter M.F. Mbithi[1,2]

1 Department of Clinical Studies, Faculty of Veterinary Medicine, University of Nairobi, Kenya

2 Office of Vice-Chancellor, University of Nairobi, Kenya

*Address all correspondence to: jamesnguhiumwangi@gmail.com

References

[1] Wanyoike MM, Wahome RG. Small-scale farming systems. In: Workshop Proceedings on Cattle Production in Kenya-Strategies for Research Planning and Implementation. December 2003 KARI HQ. Published 2004; pp. 87-133

[2] Nguhiu-Mwangi J, Mbithi PMF, Wabacha JK, Mbuthia PG. Factors associated with the occurrence of claw disorders in dairy cows under smallholder production systems in urban and peri-urban areas of Nairobi. Veterinarski Arhiv. 2008;**78**(4):343-355

[3] Nguhiu-Mwangi J, Mbithi PMF, Wabacha JK, Mbuthia PG. Prevalence of laminitis and the patterns of claw lesions in dairy cows in Nairobi and the peri-urban districts. Bulletin of Animal Health and Production in Africa. 2009;**57**:199-208

[4] Van der Tol PPJ, Metz JMH, Noordhuizen-Stassen EN, Back W, Braam CR, Weijs WA. The vertical ground reaction force and the distribution on claws of dairy cows while walking on a flat substrate. Journal of Dairy Science. 2003;**86**:2875-2883

[5] Van der Tol PPJ, Metz JMH, Noordhuizen-Stassen EN, Back W, Braam CR, Weijs WA. The force and pressure distribution on the claws of cattle and the biomechanical effect of preventive trimming. In: Proceedings of the 13th International Symposium and 5th Conference on Lameness in Ruminants; 11-15 February; Maribor, Slovenija. 2004. p. 102

[6] Nocek JE. Bovine acidosis: Implications on laminitis. Journal of Dairy Science. 1997;**80**:1005-1028

[7] Belge A, Bakir B. Subclinical laminitis in dairy cattle: 205 selected cases. Turkish Journal of Veterinary and Animal Sciences. 2005;**29**:9-15

[8] Nguhiu-Mwangi J. Characteristics of laminitis and associated claw lesions in dairy cows in Nairobi and its environs [PhD Thesis]. Nairobi, Kenya: University of Nairobi; 2007

[9] Nguhiu-Mwangi J, Mbithi PMF, Wabacha JK, Mbuthia PG. Risk (predisposing) factors from non-infectious claw disorders in dairy cows under varying zero-grazing systems. In: Perez-Marin CC, editor. A Bird's-Eye View of Veterinary Medicine. Rijeka, Croatia: InTech; 2012. pp. 393-422. DOI: 10.5772/29795.ch21. ISBN: 978-953-51-0031-7

[10] Bergsten C. Haemorrhages of the sole horn of dairy cows as a retrospective indicator of laminitis: An epidemiological study. Acta Veterinaria Scandinavica. 1994;**35**:55-66

[11] Nguhiu-Mwangi J, Mbithi PMF, Wabacha JK, Mbuthia PG. Prevalence of sole haemorrhages and its correction with subclinical and chronic laminitis in dairy cows. Bulletin of Animal Health and Production in Africa. 2007;**55**:232-242

[12] Hirschberg RM, Plendl J. Pododermal angiogenesis and angioadaptation in the bovine claw. Microscopy Research and Technique. 2005;**66**:145-155

[13] Manske T, Hultgren J, Bergsten C. The effect of claw trimming on the hoof health of Swedish dairy cattle. Preventive Veterinary Medicine. 2002;**54**:113-129

[14] Bell EL. Description of claw horn lesions and associated risk factors in dairy cattle in the Lower Fraser Valley [MSc Thesis]. British Columbia, Canada: The University of British Columbia; 2004

[15] Nguhiu-Mwangi J, Mbithi PMF, Wabacha JK, Mbuthia PG. Disorders

of the claw and their association with laminitis in smallholder zero-grazed dairy cows. International Journal of Veterinary Science and Medicine. 2017;**6**(2):64-69

[16] Newsome RF, Green MJ, Bell NJ, Bollard NJ, Mason CS, Whay HR, et al. A prospective cohort study of digital cushion and corium thickness. Part 1: Associations with body condition, lesion incidence and proximity to calving. Journal of Dairy Science. 2017;**100**:4745-4758

[17] Mülling CKW, Greenough PR. Applied physiopathology of the foot. In: Proceedings of the 14th World Buiatrics Congress; 15-19 October 2006; Nice, France. 2006. pp. 103-117

[18] Blowey R. Factors associated with lameness in dairy cattle. In Practice. 2005;**27**:154-162

[19] Knott L, Tarlton JF, Craft H, Webster AJF. Effects of housing, parturition and diet change on the biochemistry and biomechanics of the support structures of the hoof of dairy heifers. Veterinary Journal. 2007;**174**:277-287. DOI: 10.1016/j.tvjl.2006.09.007

[20] Tarlton JF, Holah DE, Evans KM, Jones S, Pearson GR, Webster AJ. Biomechanical and histopathological changes in the support structures of bovine hooves around the time of first calving. Veterinary Journal. 2002;**163**:196-204

[21] Chapinal N, de Passillé AM, Rushen J. Weight distribution and gait in dairy cattle are affected by milking and late pregnancy. Journal of Dairy Science. 2009;**92**:581-588

[22] Franck A, Cocquyt G, Simoens P, De Belie N. Biomechanical properties of bovine claw horn. Biosystems Engineering. 2006;**93**(4):459-467

[23] Somers JGCJ, Frankena K, Noordhuizen-Stassen EN, Metz JHM. Prevalence of claw disorders in Dutch dairy cows exposed to several floor systems. Journal of Dairy Science. 2003;**86**:2082-2093

[24] Vokey FJ, Guard CL, Erb HN, Galton DM. Effects of alley and stall surfaces on indices of claw and leg health in dairy cattle housed in a free-stall barn. Journal of Dairy Science. 2001;**84**:2686-2699

[25] Luna LG. Mannual of the Histological Staining Methods of the Armed Forces Institute of Pathology. 3rd ed. New York: McGraw Hill; 1968

[26] Nguhiu-Mwangi J, Mbithi PMF, Mbuthia PG. Laminitis and laminitis-associated claw conditions in smallholder zeo-grazed cows. In: Claw Disorders in Dairy Cows Under Smallholder Zero-grazing Units. Germany. ISBN: 978-3-639-66879-7, ch3: Scholars' Press, OmniScriptum GmbH & Co. KG; 2015. pp. 86-130

[27] Somers JGCJ, Schouten WGP, Frankena K, Noordhuizen-Stassen EN, Metz JHM. Development of claw traits and claw lesions in dairy cows kept on different floor systems. Journal of Dairy Science. 2005;**88**:110-120

[28] Vermunt JJ. Herd lameness: A review, major causal factors and guidelines for prevention and control. In: Proceedings of the 13th International Symposium and 5th Conference on Lameness in Ruminants; 11-15 February 2004; Maribor, Slovenija. pp. 1-15

[29] Boosman R, Nemeth F, Gruys E, Klarenbeek A. Arteriographical and pathological changes in chronic laminitis in dairy cattle. Veterinary Quarterly. 1989;**11**:144-155

[30] Maclean CW. A postmortem X-ray study of laminitis in barley beef animals. Veterinary Record. 1970;**86**:457-462

[31] Newsome R, Green MJ, Bell NJ, Chagunda MGG, Mason CS, Rutland CS, et al. Linking bone development on the caudal aspect of the distal phalanx with lameness during life. Journal of Dairy Science. 2016;**99**:4512-4525

[32] Tsuka T, Ooshita K, Sugiyama A, Osaki T, Okamoto Y, Minami S, et al. Quantitative evaluation of bone development of the distal phalanx of the cow hind limb using computed tomography. Journal of Dairy Science. 2012;**95**:127-138

[33] Greenough PR, Vermunt JJ, Mckinnon JJ, Fathy FA, Berg PA, Cohen RDH. Laminitis-like changes in the claws of feedlot cattle. Canadian Veterinary Journal. 1990;**31**:202-208

[34] Jubb KVF, Kennedy PC, Palmer N. Pathology of Domestic Animals. 3rd ed. Vol. 1. New York: Academic Press, Inc Harcourt Brace Jovanovich Publishers; 1993. pp. 61-63

[35] Russell AM, Rowlands GJ, Shaw SR, Weaver AD. Survey of lameness in British dairy cattle. Veterinary Record. 1982;**111**:155-160

[36] Tranter WP, Morris RS, Dohoo IR, Williamson NB. A case-control study of lameness in dairy cows. Preventive Veterinary Medicine. 1993;**15**:191-203

[37] Vermunt JJ, Leach DH. A scanning elcectron microscopic study of vascular system of the bovine hind limb claw. New Zealand Veterinary Journal. 1992;**40**:146-154

[38] Hirschberg R, Mülling C, Budras KD. Pododermal angioarchitecture of the bovine claw in relation to form and function of the papillary body. A scanning electron microscopic study. Microscopy Research and Technique. 2001;**54**:375-385

[39] Christmann U, Belknap EB, Lin HC, Belknap JK. Evaluation of hemodynamics in the normal and laminitic bovine digit. In: Proceedings of the 12th International Symposium on Lameness in Ruminants; 9-13 January 2002; Orlando Florida, U S A. pp. 165-166

[40] Mülling CKW, Grönemeyer D. Foot Anatomy: New Methods of Investigation and Therapeutic Implications. Paris/Frankreich: Société Francaise de Buiatrie; 2004, 2004. pp. 157-161

[41] Andersson L, Berman A. Pathology of bovine laminitis especially as regards vascular lesions. Acta Veterinaria Scandinavica. 1980;**21**:559

[42] Singh SS, Murray RD, Ward WR. Histopathological and morphometric studies on the hooves of dairy and beef cattle in relation to overgrown sole and laminitis. Journal of Comparative Pathology. 1992;**107**:319-328

[43] Bergsten C, Mülling C. Some reflections on research on bovine laminitis aspects of clinical and fundamental research. In: Proceedings of the 13th International Symposium and 5th Conference on Lameness in Ruminants; 11-15 February 2004; Maribor, Slovenija. p. 94

[44] Shearer JK, van Amstel S. Lameness in dairy cattle. In: Proceedings of 2000 Kentucky Dairy Conference. pp. 1-11

[45] Boosman R, Koeman J, Nap R. Histopatholgy of the bovine pododerm in relation to age and chronic laminitis. Zentralblatt für Veterinärmedizin. Reihe A. 1989;**36**:438-446

[46] Tarlton JF, Webster AJ. A biochemical and biomechanical basis for the pathogenesis of claw horn lesions. In: Shearer JK, editor. Proceedings of the 12th International Symposium on Lameness in Ruminants; 9-13 January 2002; Orlando Florida. pp. 395-398

Section 3

The Cardiorespiratory and Reproductive Systems

Chapter 4

Myocardial Metabolism

Dmitrii Oleinikov

Abstract

Myocardial metabolism alterations are associated with myocardial dystrophy and lead to the heart chambers dilatation, decreased contractility, organs perfusion and depended on symptoms. Nowadays heart failure treatment in veterinary medicine includes neurohormonal, circulatory and contractile aspects of this pathological state. Unfortunately, energy supplying component not presented in modern recommendations. Most of the used medications changing contractile ability, through the control of myocardial filaments sensibility to the different ions, but don't affect the ability of cardiomyocytes to produce enough energy for this work. In order to understand the heart failure syndrome more completely, we should elucidate features, characteristics, and interactions between components of myocardial energy supply.

Keywords: myocardial metabolism, insulin, insulin resistance, adropin, energy metabolism, heart failure

1. Introduction

The myocardium is one of the most energy-dependent structures. It demands about 6 kilograms of ATP per day [115]. In order to sustain an efficient energy supply, it has an advanced system producing enough ATP. In the organism, there are two ways to support this demand: production and accumulation. Accumulation is not suitable for the heart due to specific anatomy—most of the cytoplasms consist of myofibrils. According to this fact, in the adult heart, we observe low concentrations of ATP and many ATP-hydrolases. Total resynthesis of all ATP volume takes only 10 seconds in a normal myocardium [32, 55]. Most of the energy resources (~70%) are used for contraction and the rest—for ion pump function (K, Na, Ca pumps ATPases). This system is well coordinated, which helps to maintain the normal flux of energy substrates and ions.

In average, the heart consumes about 20 g of carbohydrates, 30 g of free fatty acids (FFA), and triglycerides (TG). These substrates are oxidized in 35 L of oxygen to produce ATP from ADP [171].

Oxidative phosphorylation of FFA gives about 60% of all produced ATP, while glucose, lactate, and other carbohydrates oxidation produce about 30% of all macroergic compounds. In addition, for energy supplement ketone bodies and amino acids can be utilized. Glucose utilization can be the main energy source in specific conditions (high-carbohydrate diet). Therefore, in understanding myocardial metabolic features, changes during heart failure could provide vital information for early diagnostics and therapy of myocardial diseases [99, 112].

Heart failure syndrome is a consequence of the main heart disease and associated with compensatory mechanism dysfunction, formation, and activation of pathological interactions between components of neurohumoral regulation systems [203]. Decompensation is a condition, which is always connected with reduced energy production and suppressed myocardial metabolism. For example, systolic dysfunction leads to sympathoadrenal system hyperactivation, which is associated with increased heart rate. Catecholamines activate beta-adrenergic receptors, which increase myocardial oxygen consumption due to raised FFA utilization to produce enough energy. This situation leads to increased ADP volume and negative inotropic effect, which is badly tolerated during heart failure and geometrically progress during chronic sympathetic tonus [36, 96, 115, 122, 164].

2. Metabolism in the adult healthy heart

The main substrates for ATP production are carbohydrates and free fatty acids [98]. In particular, long-chained FFA, glucose, glycogen, lactate, pyruvate, ketone bodies (acetoacetate, beta-hydroxybutyrate), and amino acids (leucine, valine, and isoleucine). These compounds are metabolized to intermediates, which enter the Krebs cycle as an acetyl-coenzyme A (ACoA) or other metabolic equivalents. During substrate utilization, the proton is generated. This proton produces an energetic gradient between mitochondrial membranes, which stimulates the oxidative chain to produce chemical energy and phosphorylate ADP to ATP [60, 61, 171, 184].

Such diversity of substrates for common energy source production predispose to several concepts: (1) myocardial metabolism is very adaptive to organism condition and substrate environment and can vary between main energy resources; unfortunately, in heart failure this flexibility is mostly lost; (2) myocardial metabolism is a self-regulated mechanism; all the intermediates of the tricarboxylic acid cycle are mediators, controlling the main metabolic path and intensity of energy production (Randle cycle); (3) metabolites can be used as components for cell structure resynthesis, and, at the same time, cellular structures could be used as an energetic substrate; (4) metabolic dysfunction and accumulation of metabolites can damage cellular proteins and change the form and function of contractile filaments; (5) myocardial metabolism is not “intracellular chemistry”; this is a functional system, which is presented with specific structure and mediator mechanisms, assessing adaptation of cardiomyocytes to environmental variations [76, 171].

Myocardial metabolism efficiency is highly dependent on pathway and substratesutilized for ATP production. There is a Kyoto Encyclopedia of Genes and Genomes (KEGG) scheme—a collectively designed map of known molecular interactions and feedback systems of energetic metabolism in the myocardium. This map made helps to understand possible ways of energy production in the myocardium and limit its activity [30, 69]. However, we should observe common features of myocardial metabolism.

In aerobic conditions, mitochondrial oxidative phosphorylation is the main source of ATP (about 90%); the rest of macroergic compounds are produced by anaerobic utilization. Mitochondrial oxidative phosphorylation produces energy due to FADH and NADH dehydration, collected from FFA beta-oxidation and, in lesser amounts, other sources. The schematic structure of metabolic interactions designed by Stanley et al. shows the main features of energy production cycles (**Figure 1**) [140].

Transport of FFA in the cardiomyocyte is presented in two ways: passive diffusion and by specific protein transporters. Long-chained FFA are diffused in the cell, metabolized in acyl-CoA, and transported to the special proteins on the mitochondrial membrane to interact with acetyl-CoA synthase. While active transport, induced by muscle contraction or insulin (Ins) action, is sustained by FATP1, FATP6,

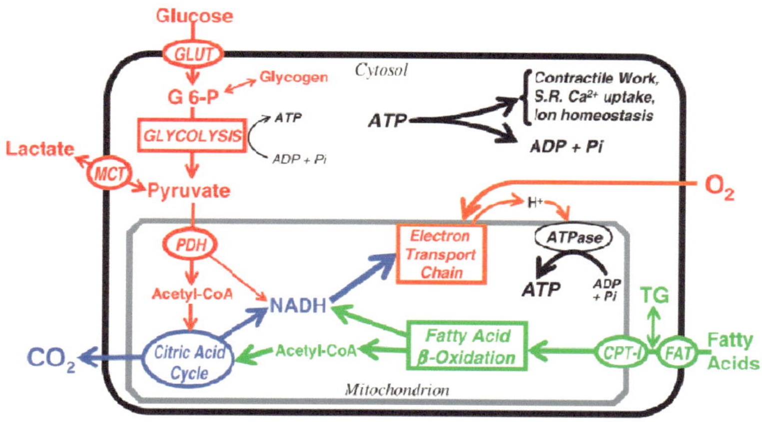

Figure 1.
Coupled metabolic reactions in the cell and mitochondria in cardiomyocyte [161]. GLUT—glucose transporter, G-6-P—glucose 6-phosphate, MCT—monocarboxylate transporter, PDH—pyruvate dehydrogenase, FAT—fatty acid membrane transporter, TG—triglyceride, and CPT-1—carnitine palmitoyltransferase 1.

and CD36 [78]. These proteins translocate FFA through the membrane, and then couple it with CoA, which is transported to lipid beta-oxidation cycle by carnitine-assosiated translocators [102].

Further, cytosolic carnitine palmitoyltransferase-1 (CPT-1) connects acyl-CoA with carnitine, forming long-chained acylcarnitine. This compound is transported with acylcarnitine translocase through the inner mitochondrial membrane and utilized in FFA beta-oxidation cycles with acetyl-CoA production. Then acetyl-CoA is metabolized in the Krebs cycle to ATP, H_2O, and CO_2. For example, in the tricarboxylic acid cycle, palmitate is oxidized with 23 moles of O_2 to produce 105 moles of ATP [63]. Nevertheless, in comparison with glucose, FFA are not effective energy sources due to their high demand for oxygen. The part of transported FFA is esterified and collected in the cytoplasm as lipid droplets (triacylglycerol-TAG) [68, 100, 101, 181]. TAG-produced ATP is about 10% of all gained ATP in physiological conditions [117]. Also, TAG is an important part of FFA oxidation, in cases when TAG-hydrolase blockade lipid beta-oxidation is severely reduced, which leads to massive lipid droplet accumulation in the cardiomyocytes [46].

The next step is activation of the Krebs cycle. This rotor starts with acetyl-CoA, collected from FFA beta-oxidation or pyruvate decarboxylation. Produced NADH and FADH2 transports are equivalent to electron chain, which stimulates ATP resynthesis in oxidative phosphorylation.

Metabolic pathways of energy production are ruled by directing components (enzymes) and feedback connection (substrate-final product). The mitochondria can bear high-energy demand states, increasing oxygen consumption almost on 85% from the basal level. This ability is very important due to the fact that most of the time it consumes only 25% of the oxidative capacity [111]. Therefore, activation/inhibition of enzymatic systems can control ATP synthesis, and, due to feedback, can correct energetic substrates, in cases of increased metabolites collection or regulation disorders. This kind of metabolic flexibility is very useful in myocardial diseases, associated or modulated by energy resources depletion and absence [31, 32].

In addition, in normal conditions myocardium utilizes lactate, which metabolizes to pyruvate by lactate dehydrogenase and gets involved in the Krebs cycle. In cases of metabolic disorders, the myocardium starts to excrete lactate in the bloodstream. This way appears when there is oxygen deficiency and the energy has to be produced by anaerobic glycolysis (ischemia, terminal stages of cardiomyopathies)

[6, 47, 104, 162]. The main transporter controlling excretion and consumption of lactate is the monocarboxylate transporter (MCT). This family consists of four subclasses, in the myocardium only 1 form of MCT-1 is presented. Also, they take a part in ketone body transport [40, 50, 64].

Glycolysis is another coexisting pathway for energy production. The first step of glycolysis starts with glucose transport through the cell membrane by the specific transporter (GLUT). In the cytoplasm glucose is metabolized to pyruvate, which is transported to the mitochondrial matrix by pyruvate dehydrogenase (PDH). Pyruvate is transformed to acetyl-CoA and gets involved to the Krebs cycle [61, 162].

The GLUT family includes 12 classes; the most important for myocardial metabolism are GLUT 1 and GLUT 4, which supplies glucose in the cardiomyocytes. GLUT 4 is insulin dependent and plays a significant role in insulin resistance formation; GLUT 1 is weakly insulin dependent; it is the source of basal glucose transport for myocytes; in addition, it could be additively recruited from cytosol in stress conditions [167]. GLUT 1 is mostly located on the sarcolemma, while GLUT 4 also attenuated to T-tubules, which is useful for "deep" glucose transport during raised energy demand and exercises. In normal conditions GLUT 1 protein expression is higher due to persisting glucose demand as an energy source. GLUT 4 concentration in the myocardium and muscle is almost equal, which means that developing insulin resistance of different etiologies leads to decreased glucose flux both in the skeletal muscle and in the myocardium. GLUT 4 is the main glucose transporter to the muscle cell, but in experiments with GLUT 4 knockout, animals show that glucose can be translocated to the myocyte by different mechanisms [34, 196].

After transport into the cell, glucose was converted to glucose-6-phosphate (G6P) by cytosolic hexokinase 2 (HX2), and then it was utilized in glycolytic reactions or stored as glycogen. Phosphofructokinases—glycolytic enzymes—which irreversibly convert G6P to fructose-6-phosphate, forming fructose-1 and 6-bisphosphate and dephosphorylating ATP to ADP. These kinases are limiting threshold for glycolytic activity and depending on ATP, AMP, citrate concentrations, and pH [131].

After glucose is converted to pyruvate, its metabolism trifurcates to lactate conversion, decarboxylation to acetyl-CoA, and carboxylation to malate or oxaloacetate. Decarboxylation is an irreversible process, catalyzed by pyruvate dehydrogenase (PDH). PDH activation is closely connected with cytosolic Ca^{+2} and Mg^{+2} concentrations, sympathetic tonus, while inhibition depends on FFA concentration in the environment. PDH is a multienzyme complex, consisting of two main parts: pyruvate dehydrogenase itself and pyruvate dehydrogenase kinase assessing pyruvate utilization. Pyruvate consumption increases in cases of decreased FAA utilization or artificial inhibition of lipid beta-oxidation. FFA and glucose turnovers in the mitochondria are controlled by the Randle cycle, and by its ways, we could admit that PDH activity is determined depending on the substrate environment (**Figure 2**) [106, 107, 137, 138].

The lactate-lactate dehydrogenase-pyruvate system is made for additive pyruvate production in cases of high demand or its discharge to lactate when the FFA wing is activated in Randle's cycle. In heart failure, FAA consumption is increased due to adrenergic hyperactivation and compensatory mechanisms; this leads to PDH inhibition, and glucose metabolites are converted to lactate, instead of pyruvate, and eliminated to the bloodstream. This causes lactate and pyruvate depletion in the cytosol; the relative lactate/pyruvate ration raises and negatively influences energy supplementation for submembrane structures, which control ion recirculation [20, 98, 121, 136, 153].

The final step of glucose utilization is an oxidation of acetyl-CoA to CO_2 in the Krebs cycle and formation of 31 ATP molecules. Due to produced ATP amounts, oxidative glycolysis is the most effective energy source.

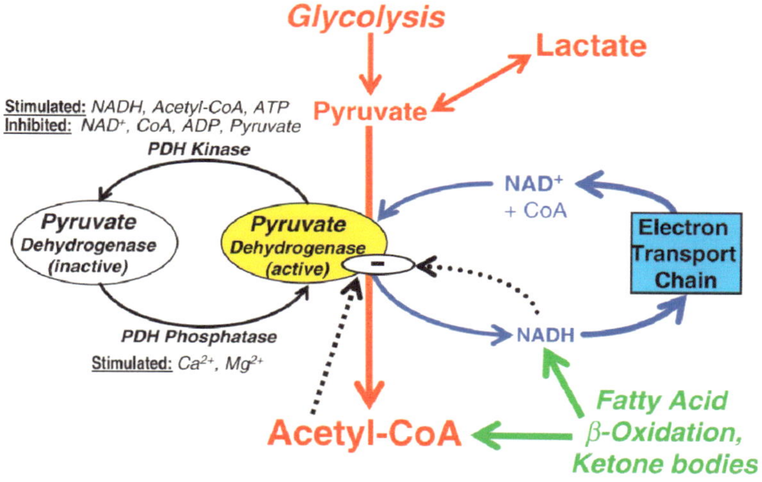

Figure 2.
Pyruvate metabolism in normal myocardium (Stanley et al., 2002).

It should be noted that such intermediates as G6P and lactate can also be metabolized in alternative ways. G6P can be utilized in the pentose phosphate pathway (PPP), producing NADH in association with O_2 or a pentose (substrate for nucleotides) in a hypoxic environment. In addition, G6P can be converted to sorbitol, uridine diphosphate-N-acetylglucosamine, which can provide O-associated glycosylation of contractile filaments and Ca^{+2} ion pumps of the sarcoplasmic reticulum (SR). In cases of massive protein glycosylation, the cell can undergo apoptosis [6, 56, 80, 141].

The intensity of FFA utilization by a healthy myocardium depends on the concentration of non-esterified FFA in the blood, the activity of metabolism modulation mediators (catecholamine, thyroxin, triiodothyronine, insulin, cortisol, adropin) can be increased four times during the day. FFA are transported to cardiomyocytes in non-esterified form, bound with albumin or as chylomicrons, lipoproteins, and then they translocated in the cytoplasm and oxidized. FFA releases are depended on catecholamine-induced activation of hormone-dependent lipase [195]. Therefore, FFA plasma level significantly increased in cases of adrenergic activation, insulin depletion, insulin resistance, hypothyroid condition, hyperadrenocorticism, etc. [98, 128, 201].

In addition, FFA myocardial metabolism is also influenced by secondary messenger, AMP-activated protein kinase (AMPK), which activity is closely connected with the AMP/ATP ratio in the cytosol. This molecule has several actions: (1) AMPK inhibits malonyl-CoA production, switching off acetyl-CoA-synthase, leading to decreased FFA cytosol accumulation; (2) ongoing decrease of malonyl-CoA inhibits bounding of CPT-1 and stimulates transport of acetyl-CoA to the mitochondria for oxidation; and (3) AMPK stimulates expression of FATP and CD36 on cardiomyocyte outer membranes [68, 100, 101, 181].

It should be mentioned that peroxisome proliferator-activated receptor-alpha (PPAR-a) is also a regulator of FFA oxidation. This receptor is a part of ligand-activated family of nuclear receptors. Ligands of the FFA receptor, in active form PPAR-a, activate the synthesis of lipid beta-oxidation enzymes [59]. In experiments, it was observed that this receptor deactivation leads to decreasing FFA oxidation capacity in cardiomyocytes, due to significant depletion of lipid oxidation enzymes. During ischemia and insulin resistance in diabetic mice, induced by streptozotocin, PPAR-a knockout animals were more stable in the ischemia–reperfusion protocol, than the control group mice. This can be explained by the fact that the inhibition of FFA oxidative utilization promotes glycolysis. Inactivated PPAR-a allows to perform increased oxidative glycolysis (decreased FFA oxidation in the Randle cycle), improve GLUT 4 translocation and PDH activation, and improve the severity of insulin resistance. In cases of hypoxic ischemia, this will give a chance for cardiomyocytes' survival due to glycolysis and energy production. In addition, increased PPAR-a expression promotes GLUT 4 genes suppression, leading to insulin resistance and, indirectly, stimulates FFA oxidation metabolites accumulation, this inhibits glycolysis wing of the Randle cycle, decreases GLUT 4 trafficking activity, and suppresses insulin receptor sensitivity due to PI-3-kinase inhibition [33, 127].

However, in cases of active oxidation in tricarboxylic acid cycle with high production of malonyl-CoA, normal transport of FFA to the mitochondrial inner membrane is stopped. Also, membrane translocation of lipids is inhibited by insulin [28, 72].

Utilization of amino acids (predominately leucine, valine, and isoleucine) in energy metabolism is less effective than glycolysis and FFA beta-oxidation. Active amino acid utilization leads to metabolite accumulation; this state is associated with cardiomyopathies and respiratory chain damage in the mitochondria. Metabolism of this substrate is associated with ketoacid formation; part of them could be converted to acetyl-CoA and used in the Krebs cycle [145].

Another substrate are ketone bodies (beta-hydroxybutyrate and acetoacetate). These compounds are produced by the liver during FFA oxidation, and under normal conditions, their level in the plasma is very low, and so they do not actively utilize in myocardial energy metabolism. However, lipomobilization and insulin depletion (diabetes mellitus) could be exceptions for this situation; this condition leads to decreased glycolysis and lactate consumption by cardiomyocytes. In addition, ketone body utilization inhibits FFA oxidation, altering the process of dissociation of acetyl- CoA to free CoA. This complex promotes secondary to heart failure often noted in patients with diabetes mellitus [49, 95, 160].

In experimental models, it was noted that ketone utilization inhibits lactate oxidation for 30–60% and palmitate for 22%. Later, in vivo experiments admitted that parallel administration of FFA and hydroxybutyrate markedly inhibits FFA oxidation in pigs. It has to be noted that the levels of malonyl-CoA and acetyl-CoA were unchanged. In a similar experiment, it was shown that high concentration of ketone bodies promotes the Krebs cycle blockade and downregulates contractility of cardiomyocytes. So, ketones could be energy substrate to the myocardium, but it blocks other more useful ways of energy production, due to significant demand for oxygen [160, 173].

Some intercellular conditions can influence on metabolism intensity and oxidative potential. The significant parameter of the functional condition of the cell is redox potential. Pyridine compounds (NAD, NADH, NADP, NADPH) play the most important role in this state. One of the simplest estimations of redox potential in a cell is cytoplasmic and mitochondrial NAD/NADH ratio. It is considered that NAD depletion and NADH raise characterize inhibition of oxidation in the mitochondria and slowing of Krebs cycle. This was also noted during hypoxia, enzyme defects, and lack of energy substrates [93].

There are complexes of cytoplasmic oxidoreductase enzymes dependent on NAD concentration. The most active one is lactate dehydrogenase (LDH). LDH, depending on the intracellular environment, can produce NAD and lactate from pyruvate, or reverse this reaction to produce pyruvate and NADH. There are many malate dehydrogenases (MDH) in the mitochondria, which is the part of the malate–aspartate shuttle. In particular, MDH catalyzes the metabolism of oxaloacetate and NADH to malate and NAD, and then malate is transported to the mitochondria, while the NAD/NADH ratio increased in the cytoplasm. In addition,

MDH takes part in nitrogen metabolism, rarely can be activated to produce energy from aspartate [12, 67, 85, 146].

High NAD/NADH ratio promotes normal substrate oxidation and saves redox potential to sustain electron transport in oxidative metabolism. As already been said, LDH and glyceraldehyde 3-phosphate dehydrogenase (GAPDH) both use NAD/NADH as a cofactor. GAPDH produces NADH, which is oxidized to NAD by LDH. In anaerobic conditions, both of these enzymes produce NAD, which is utilized in glycolysis. In the aerobic state, NADH reoxidation is connected with its utilization in the mitochondrial respiratory chain. Due to impermeability of mitochondrial membranes to NAD and NADH, there are several shuttles for NADH transport and NAD resynthesis. Discussed above, the malate–aspartate shuttle is predominant in the myocardium [55, 118].

Increased ATP consumption promotes oxidative phosphorylation and increases NAD/NADH ratio. This condition activates several NAD-dependent enzymes: isocitrate dehydrogenase, alpha-ketoglutarate dehydrogenase, and MDH which increase the Krebs cycle intensity [163, 189].

3. Regulation of carbohydrates and FFA oxidation

The main regulator of carbohydrates oxidation is FFA utilization. Increased FFA consumption leads to its intermediate accumulation, which blocks PDH. At the same time, decreased FFA consumption promotes glycolysis and lactate oxidation, due to citrate, NADH, and acetyl-CoA deficiency in the mitochondrial matrix. The last part is often noted in cardiomyopathies and during ischemia [54, 161].

Modern researches showed an impressive role of small molecule proteins—energy homeostasis regulators. Of course, there are many molecules and factors that control energy metabolism, one stimulates appetite (ghrelin, galanin, neuropeptide Y) and another is an anorexigenic (leptin, nesfatin-1) [71, 155]. The first found molecule, which regulates energetic homeostasis, was insulin (Ins); its action was first noted as neurogenic appetite suppression. Later leptin was found—hormone, produced by adipose tissue—and elucidates general adipose tissue state [199]. Then ghrelin and nesfatin-1 were found, with antagonist action to leptin effects on adipose tissue [77, 120]. On the next decades, there was intensive research in the field of lipid homeostasis and appetite-controlling peptides. Many molecules were found; the most important are preptin, irisin, and adropin.

Insulin (Ins) is a hormone with a huge specter of physiological influence, but in this papers, we discuss only three effects: on heart pump function, on Ca^{+2} ion circulation, and as a mediator between cell communication. Ins-induced transport of glucose is the main mechanism of energy production of membrane-associated ATPases and ion pumps. Controlling pump function, Ins indirectly influences cytoplasmic concentration and equilibration of Ca^{+2}; it mediates cascades of reactions to stimulate Ca consumption or excretion. Ins is involved in endothelial function, regulating NO production and tissue perfusion (including coronary vessels). And, of course, it influences on the contractile ability of cardiomyocytes due to energy metabolism modulation.

As an indirect effect, abilities of Ins to control the availability of energy substrates (effects on liver and adipose tissue) and tissue perfusion should be noted. Ins inhibits TG hydrolysis in adipose tissue (depressing lipomobilizating hormones), decreasing the level of circulating FFA. In addition, reactive Ins secretion increases tissue perfusion due to blood vessels smooth muscle relaxation. This effect plays a significant role during exercise, hypertension, and acute and chronic heart failure [70, 136, 165].

Direct Ins action regulates key enzymes (6-phosphofructokinase 1 and 2, glycogen phosphorylase and synthase, PDH, hormone-dependent lipase, acetyl-CoA carboxylase) and transporters (GLUT family, CPT-1, CD36/FAPT). Interactions between main metabolic substrates (glucose and FFA) are elucidated by Randle's cycle [136]. Transmembrane glucose transport by GLUT 1 and GLUT 4 is modulated by Ins (both transporters are Ins-determined, but GLUT 1 is less dependent). GLUT 4 is significantly presented in myocardium tissue; this helps to sustain myocardial energy flexibility in exercises and heart failure. Ins influence on glycogen accumulation in several ways: decreasing glucose utilization (FFA oxidation predominance, leads to PDH blockade, glucose intermediates converted to glycogen); HX2 converting capacity in overloaded glucose transport (Ins-dependent GLUT 4 exocytosis); glycogen utilization in glucose depletion. It should be mentioned that glycogen is oxidized more actively, than glucose, due to its already intracellular location and production of more ATP. In addition, Ins stimulates glycogen synthase directly and through G6P raise [52, 86]. Ins and PDH interactions are not clear. We should consider the effects of FFA oxidation suppression (decreased acetyl-CoA concentration in mitochondria), influence on PDH phosphatase, NAD/NADH ratio, and Ca^{+2} concentration. Generally, Ins is controlling glycolysis indirectly by metabolite and substrate availability and directly through enzymatic systems (mentioned above). Ins' influence on FFA oxidation is closely connected with its effects on glycolysis and partly described above. By the way, Ins suppresses CPT-1 function, due to malonyl-CoA concentration. It can be explained by the fact that malonyl-CoA is produced by acetyl-CoA carboxylase, which is in direct control of Ins [57, 58].

Mediator effect of Ins between cells is described by its effects on PDH, HX2, phosphofructokinase, glycogen synthase, acetyl-CoA carboxylase, hormone-dependent lipase, PDH kinase, MAP kinase, and lactate intercellular shuttle and based on metabolic influence.

As for leptin, its effects were observed in recent research of dogs with chronic degenerative valve disease. In the experiment the raise of circulating leptin and leptin microRNA in this disease was noted. Observed dogs were not suffering from obesity, so found leptin changes are connected with heart failure syndrome. In addition, the correlation between leptin level and heart failure severity was found [45].

Preptin is a hormone modulating carbohydrate metabolism; it is a part of the insulin family (as insulin, insulin-like growth factor-1, proinsulin-like factor-2, relaxin-2). In experiments, it was found that it is secreted together with insulin and promotes glucose utilization in insulin-like ways. There was a strong connection between preptin expression and insulin resistance. Generally, this hormone plays a role in hepatic glycogenesis and bone density (osteoclasts proliferation) and modulates sensitivity to insulin and adaptation to energetic substrates [1, 10, 126, 186].

Adropin is a recently found hormone controlling lipid metabolism. Adropin regulates energy metabolism, depending on the diet type (significantly raised on a high-fat diet). Systemic administration of adropin decreases hepatosteatosis and hyperinsulinemia severity (moderating carbohydrate-FFA metabolism in peripheral tissues). In researches, a connection between heart failure severity and circulating adropin concentration (high severity of heart failure-high adropin level) was noted. Also in insulin resistance, the level of circulating adropin is decreased and correlated with atherosclerosis risks in diabetes mellitus. Low levels of adropin were associated with endothelial dysfunction and high risk of heart X syndrome. Adropin suppresses the activity of PDH kinase 4, which promotes normal pyruvate utilization in Krebs cycle and decreases CPT-1 activity and traffic of CD36 transporters, decreasing FFA transport in cardiomyocytes. The main functions of adropin consist of regulating NO availability, decreasing lipogenic gene expression, decreasing dyslipidemia and hepatic steatosis, modifying insulin resistance and glucose tolerance, and controlling metabolic homeostasis [37–39, 82, 91, 168].

Irisin is a hormone controlling the conversion of white to brown adipose tissue. The white adipose tissue has a lack of mitochondria and lots of TG and FFA and produces leptin, ghrelin, nesfatin-1 [15, 27, 135, 178]. While the brown adipose tissue contains lots of mitochondria and lipid droplets. In this cell, high amounts of uncoupling protein-1 are presented. This protein promotes uncoupling of ATP production from FFA oxidation, instead of ADP phosphorylation, and produces heat [62]. In experiments, it was noted that high amounts of circulating irisin are presented in cases of obesity, which can be characterized as irisin resistance (insulin resistance-like) [166]. Irisin is predominantly synthesized in skeletal muscles during exercises. The main actions of this hormone are toward decreasing of white adipose tissue, controlling temperature homeostasis, increasing of glucose tolerance, decreasing obesity, and modulating insulin resistance [144, 198].

Besides, there are also biologically active molecules, which have paracrine effects. This molecule does not affect myocardial metabolism by itself, but promoting reactions could affect the contractile ability of cardiomyocytes. Among them are cytokines, thrombocyte-activating factor (TAF), reactive oxygen species (ROS), arachidonic acid, and nitrogen oxide (NO). The sources of these peptides are the cardiomyocyte itself, endotheliocytes, and migrating immune cells (mononuclear phagocytes, lymphocytes, etc.) [159].

Cytokines include TNF-a, IL-1, and IL-6. TNF-a is produced in cardiomyocytes during injury; the most effects of this peptide are described in ischemia–reperfusion syndrome, due to its significant negative inotropic effect. The main promoters of TNF-a production are hypoxia and ROS. Negative inotropic effect development is staged. First, immediately after the injury, sphingosine is produced from sphingomyelin, which inhibits RyR2 receptors of SR and decreases Ca^{+2}-dependent Ca^{+2} release, suppressing contractility. In parallel, direct cytotoxic effect developed, due to mitochondrial oxidation uncoupling. And then, NO-dependent Ca^{+2} transport suppression is developed. Produced NO-superoxide promotes contractile filament damage and cardiomyocyte apoptosis [2, 43, 105, 123, 148].

Interleukins are the main inflammatory mediators; their action closely interacted with TNF-a, developing NO release, suppression of Ca^{+2} turn over regulation genes and decreasing cAMP in cardiomyocytes [41, 42, 74, 179].

Thrombocyte-activating factor (TAF) is a phosphoglyceride with a potent pro-inflammatory effect. This cytokine is produced by cardiomyocytes, endotheliocytes, and histiocytes. TAF pathological effects are associated with significant vasoconstriction, contractility decrease, ROS, and superoxide release and autolysis activation [35, 48].

Arachidonic acid and its metabolites is part of membrane phospholipids in cardiomyocytes, but in case of injury, these compounds are degraded by phospholipase A2, which is high Ca^{+2} concentration-dependent. Arachidonic metabolites damage ionic channels components, receptors, intercalated disks and provoke cytoplasmic acidosis, Ca^{+2} hyperaccumulation [192].

Adenosine is a metabolite of adenine nucleotide; it has a wide specter of action: coronary artery dilatation, negative chronotropic, dromotropic, and inotropic effects by means of A1 and A2 receptors. Adenosine is also a catecholamine antagonist (decreases cAMP activity), stimulates protein kinase C (PKC), promotes macroergic compounds restoration, and inhibits some ROS and neutrophils activity [88, 157].

PKC is a part of intracellular myocardial metabolism regulation. This kinase is sensitive to Ca^{+2} cytoplasm accumulation, angiotensin II, phenylephrine, and endothelin stimulation. As a response to this stimulation, PKC downregulates troponin; sensitivity of troponin to Ca^{+2} promotes myofibrillar disruption and decreases contractile ability, fibrosis, and hypertrophy of cardiomyocytes. In experiments, it was noted that increased PKC expression provokes myocardial hypertrophy and fetal metabolic genotype activation and significantly alters Ca^{+2} ion transmembrane circulation [7, 185, 187]. This can be explained by decreased SERCA2 and phospholamban protein expression, suppression of Na/CA and Na/H ionic pumps, PKC-dependent phosphorylation of the myofilament and troponin proteins, and downregulation of Ca^{+2}-dependent membrane transporters, which indirectly negatively influence on energy metabolism [174].

CaMKK II—calmodulin-dependent kinase— is activated by Ca^{+2} accumulation in the cytoplasm. CaMKK II independently or by AMPK stimulation promotes GLUT 4 trafficking and exocytosis. In experiments a compound stimulation of GLUT 4 exocytosis and its retention on the outer part of the cell membrane by AMP, PKC, and CaMKK II was elucidated. By these means, muscle contraction promotes GLUT 4 exocytosis and glucose transport, but in cases of pathologic Ca^{+2} cytoplasm accumulation, GLUT 4 could not move into the cell, which alters glucose consumption and promotes increasing of FFA utilization (Randle cycle). Catecholamine-induced tachycardia provokes altered GLUT 4 endocytosis, insulin resistance, and glycolysis inhibition [90].

As already been said, there are many regulating mediators. However, Ca^{+2} ions can influence myocardial metabolism by themselves. The raise of Ca cytoplasmic concentration (SR release) is determined by the following mechanisms: Ca^{+2}-dependent Ca^{+2} release (calcium sparks), SR depolarization, pH changes, voltage-dependent changes of T-tubules and triad membranes, and inositol-dependent release. Calcium provokes GLUT 4 exocytosis and increases glucose consumption. First, this effect was described in experiments with caffeine influence on cardiomyocytes. Myocytes began to utilize glucose, while being incubated with low caffeine concentration.

Nitric oxide decreases cardiomyocyte utilization of glucose due to cGMP effects. In experiments, it was noted that NO-synthase blockade promotes stabilization of ischemic myocardium metabolic state. Some researchers pointed at fact that cGMP and glucose metabolism are not connected, so the real influence of No on metabolism is not clear, but its effects should be noted. In addition, NO has a negative inotropic effect in inhibiting Ca-channel and producing superoxide (peroxynitrite) [17–19, 83, 170, 197].

4. Energy substrates and contractility

Muscle contraction is a multifactor process, including energy status changes (ATP/AMP ratio variation), increased intercellular Ca^{+2} accumulation, stretch, GLUT 4 exocytosis, glucose and FFA consumption, etc.

Many types of research showed the high effectiveness of myocardial contractility in conditions of intensive glucose utilization, and, at the same time, increased FFA consumption on 26% did not promote equal raise in contractility, but only oxygen demand raised [109, 154]. Target disabling FFA oxidation reactions and FFA bounding to not available compounds decreases oxygen demand and increases the mechanic power of rat's heart contraction. Combination of insulin and glucose promotes to decrease the heart's oxygen demand to 39% [79]. These effects are not clearly understood because theoretically palmitate or oleate utilization need fewer molecules of O_2 to produce one molecule of ATP in comparison with glucose or lactate. A possible explanation is connected with interactions between long-chained FFA and Ca^{+2} channels (increases ATP demand for a pump ATP-ase) [75, 109, 154].

Recent studies showed that increased concentration of FFA and TG in the cytoplasm can provoke lipotoxicity in the myocardium, presented in neutral lipids and ceramides accumulation, leading to cell's apoptosis and decreased contractility. In experiments, Zhou showed that in the diabetic rat, high rates of TG and ceramides were accumulated, promoting DCM-phenotype changes, decreased contractility, and high indexes of cardiomyocytes apoptosis. Nevertheless, in the case of troglitazone, the manifestation of the FFA block mentioned significantly decreased. By this time lipid-induced myocardium remodeling is still mostly unknown, but this process could be associated with cell apoptosis, decreased contractility due to intensive FFA utilization and significantly depressed glycolysis [53, 108, 125, 150, 151, 156, 158, 180, 194, 195].

Heart failure syndrome, despite etiology, development is always associated with an energy deficit. During this state individual cardiomyocytes are under the increased workload associated with the high demand for macroergic substrates, but their production is severely depleted. This state is so-called an engine out of fuel due to decreased amounts of creatine phosphate and ATP [115]. Compensatory and pathological cardiomyocyte hypertrophy is associated with decreased creatine phosphate/ATP ratio, and later ATP decreases too. The creatine phosphate/ATP ratio is a reliable prognostic marker in heart failure worsening [114].

5. Myocardial metabolism in heart failure

Developing heart failure leads to decreased flexibility of myocardial metabolism. On the certain stages, HF has a tendency to switch FFA utilization as the main energy substrate to glucose oxidation. Decreased FFA consumption, depleted FFA oxidation enzymes, and mitochondrial oxidation biomarkers characterize this stage. This switch is usually early noted. In experiments, it was admitted that metabolic changes in rat myocardium are found in the second week after artificial aortic constriction, while decreased contractility presented only on the 20th week after bandage [24]. Some researchers say that glycolysis predomination is a marker of terminal myocardial metabolism dysfunction. These changes are associated with adaptation because glycolysis demands 12% less oxygen to produce same the amounts of ATP, then FFA oxidation [3, 79].

Transition to glycolysis promotes increased glucose consumption and raised GLUT 1 expression. In parallel, glucose oxidation is also altered, which leads to uncoupling of glycolysis and glucose oxidation. The combination of depressed FFA utilization and glucose oxidation shows decreased mitochondrial oxidative potential ГЛЮТ1 [87, 110].

During glycolysis and glucose oxidation uncoupling, due to PDH inhibition by PDK, pyruvate is not transported to the mitochondria but metabolized to lactate by LDH. This leads to cellular acidosis, and, by the way, this anaerobic glucose utilization gives only two molecules of ATP (while aerobic—32) [103]. Described changes promote cardiomyocyte hypertrophy, energy metabolism depression, ionic pump dysfunction, Ca^{+2} accumulation, decreased contractility, apoptosis, and fibrosis. It should be noted that this pattern of myocardial dysfunction development is the same for all cardiomyocytes; even in cases of pulmonary hypertension and compensatory hypertrophy of the right heart, metabolic alterations will be identical to the changes observed in the left heart failure [129].

In available data is also admitted that heart failure promotes myocardial tissue insulin resistance, partially due to neurohormonal remodeling, and is an independent predictive factor of sudden heart death in humans [23, 116]. Insulin resistance leads to decreased glucose utilization and ATP production [116, 169]. In some data, it was elucidated that the TG accumulation in muscles (found by 1H NMR method) promotes insulin resistance [81]. The dependence between TG accumulation and insulin resistance is explained by Randle' cycle: high FFA intracellular accumulation promotes raised acetyl-CoA/CoA and NADH/NAD ratios, which inhibits PDH and leads to citrate accumulation and phosphofructokinase inhibition. Associated G6P accumulation inhibits HX2, promoting intracellular glucose accumulation and decreasing intracellular glucose transport.

Insulin resistance also can be associated with high circulating insulin concentrations. Adrenergic hyperactivity, concomitant to heart failure, leads to increased glucose mobilization, hormone circulation, and insulin synthesis, lipomobilization due to catecholamines (noradrenaline). Insulin stimulates GLUT 4 and CD36 exocytosis, on the first stages it helps to produce enough ATP from glycolysis and oxidative phosphorylation. But insulin receptors have variable action mechanism. Insulin receptors have two places of connection for insulin. One of them has high affinity to hormone and promotes fast response to insulin stimulation; another is a "slow" one and is activated in cases of high insulin concentration and due to geometrical conformation partially blocks the "fast" part of the receptor. In general, insulin resistance is based on the blockade of all "fast" receptors, increased insulin concentration, and fixation of the hormone on "slow" locus of the insulin receptor [9, 11, 13, 14, 94, 116, 152, 175, 190]. Also, a high concentration of circulating FFA decreases insulin-stimulated GLUT 4 translocation. This can be explained by inhibition of Pi 3 kinase of IR-1, which phosphorylation is decreased by TG and phospholipid (FFA-acetyl-CoA, diacylglycerol, ceramides) accumulation in the cytoplasm [26]. GLUT 1 increased expression also takes a part in this process. Increased glucose flux from GLUT 1 promotes decreased GLUT 4 exocytosis and increased GLUT 4 tissue concentration. Developing GLUT 4 function reduction pathological cardiomyocyte hypertrophy and systolic dysfunction occurs [92, 177, 188]. Another factor is pyruvate utilization in anaplerotic reactions, which leads to decreased acetyl-CoA production for Kreb's cycle, glycolysis and oxidative phosphorylation uncoupling, and PDK 4 activation (promotes inhibition of insulin-stimulated glycolysis) [133].

Also it should be noted that in diabetes and insulin resistance, HX2 activity is decreased. In cell culture experiments, it was found that insulin is HX2 gene expression and protein resynthesis regulator. So, the severity of insulin resistance is a suppressor of HX2 function, leading to G6P accumulation and cytoplasm protein glycosylation. It should be admitted that decreased HX2 microRNA is associated with GLUT 4 genes and protein depletion. These interactions between insulin, HX2, and GLUT can be controlled by insulin sensibilization—by thiazolidinediones (pioglitazone, troglitazone) [124, 132].

Often heart failure is accompanied by all energy-producing enzyme dysfunction. Significant reduction of activity is noted in creatine kinase (CK) function. This enzyme regulates transfer between ATP and creatine. CK is a dimer and consists of two parts M and B, and there are three isoforms: MM, BB, MB, and mitochondrial-CK [193]. MM-CK is closely connected with SR and coupled with Ca^{+2}-ATPase, producing energy for Ca^{+2} circulation [182]. Mitochondrial-CK is located on the inner membrane of the mitochondria and works with the ADP-ATP translocator. Produced ATP is transported by translocator to mitochondrial-CK and further to creatine phosphate or ADP. This compartment distribution provides effective control of local ATP/ADP ratio and promotes mitochondrial ATP production (decreased ratio) or increases enzymes activity. But in conditions of cardiomyopathy, the normal compartment system is altered. Decompartmentalization leads to uncoupling of the mitochondria—mitochondrial-CK-ATP and phosphocreatine interactions [29, 176].

One experimental research elucidated CK activity in rats with induced heart failure. General CK activity was decreased to 45% from normal value; in particular, the most damaged was mitochondrial isoenzyme (activity was suppressed to 17% of normal). This depletion is connected with mitochondrial dysfunction. Effectiveness of mitochondrial oxygen utilization was experimentally evaluated by ADP concentration changes in presence of creatine. During this experiment, the point of ADP concentration where oxygen utilization does not raise independently to increasing APD was noted. And this level was significantly lower in the heart failure group, but at the same time, the oxidative activity of mitochondria was raised up to 30% higher than in the control group. This data shows inhibition of mitochondrial-CK function, also, indirectly, can show that mitochondrial population is decreased, but its oxidative function is upregulated [184].

CK and mitochondria interactions are very complicated and not only functional but also structural. In the cell, the mitochondria forms a crystal-like structure, predisposed to effectively produce energy sources and preserve contractility. Due to the partial isolation of the mitochondria, the contractile function is controlled by small compartments, surrounding each sarcomere and named "Intracellular Energetic Unit" (IEU). One of the most important roles in this system is played by CK isoenzymes (see above). But destructuration of this compartment will lead to substrate supplementation uncoupling and energy starvation [25, 44, 66, 183].

Heart failure is associated with morphological changes in the mitochondria: size reduction, number increase, edema, cristae deformation, homogenization, and IEU damage. The severity of mitochondrial matrix loss is correlated with heart failure stage, and, in addition, mitochondria size variability characterizes respiratory chain damage [4, 65].

Also, the mitochondria serves as controller of Ca^{+2} homeostasis in the cytoplasm. The mitochondria regulates Ca-dependent signaling by the means of ion accumulation and energy supplementation for ion pumps, producing an ionic gradient between membranes. The mitochondria directly (SERCA) or indirectly (Na/K pumps) control Ca^{+2} circulation [16, 119]. Decreased ATP synthesis promotes free Mg^{+2} accumulation, and its competing effect blocks Ca-dependent Ca release from SR [84]. Then Ca and Na accumulates due to increased activity of Na/H and Na/Ca^{+2} pumps, provoking acidosis in cardiomyocytes and decreased buffering ability of the mitochondria [200]. Usually, free Mg^{+2} concentration is low in the cytoplasm, because it is mostly bounded to ATP, but during ATP loss Mg-ion amounts raise. In this way, we can assume that increased intracellular concentration of free Mg^{+2} is a marker of decreased energy production.

In cases of ATP depletion or oxidative phosphorylation alterations, acidosis is developing. This condition promotes NA accumulation due to activation of Na/H cotransporter. Then inhibition of Na/K pump occurs. While Na accumulates in the cytoplasm, Na/Ca^{+2} exchange pump activates provoking pathological Ca^{+2} storage in the cytoplasm, mitochondrial membrane depolarization, and its inability for ionic excess buffering. This condition is predisposing to the accelerated Ca turnover and associated arrhythmias [200].

In general, switching from FFA oxidation to glycolysis during HF characterizes changing of adult heart metabolic pattern to fetal type [97]. This condition leads to disturbances in energy metabolism component gene expression. In experimental models of HF, isogenies, which switched from adult to fetal type, were sequenced [8, 149]. This fetal genotype activation promotes myocardial hypertrophy. One study analyzed 13 metabolism regulating components and expression of the atrial natriuretic peptide (ANP) and heavy beta-myosin chains (beta-MHC) in a normal adult, fetal heart, and in heart failure [139]. The ANP was upregulated in fetal and failing heart, but in HF ANP was not bound to fetal gene overexpression. Stretch, adrenergic hyperactivation, and tachycardia were the reasons for increased ANP in failing heart [147]. Beta-MHC expression was predominant in all three groups in comparison with alpha-MHC. Beta-MHC isogenies were downregulated in fetal and failing hearts, but this is connected with myofilament reduction [51, 73]. Alpha-MHC was reduced by more than 30% in both groups in comparison with the adult heart. These changes are explained by less beta-MHC oxygen and energy demand, but its contractility is also low. In addition, in fetal and failing hearts, FFA oxidation enzymes genes were also suppressed [51, 113, 143].

Fetal genotype is conditioned by hypoxic conditions during embryogenesis, and glycolysis is predominating, while after birth energy metabolism is switched to FFA oxidation. In conditions of pathologic hypertrophy, cardiomyocytes again switched to fetal metabolism in order to survive in the hypoxic environment and energy starvation. In cases of hypertension, this switch appears earlier than in cardiomyopathy [172].

In the adult heart GLUT 4 microRNA expression is rising, while GLUT 1 is decreasing in comparison with fetal heart. In the heart, failure version is observed. The same changes were endured by PDK2, PDK 4, and glycogen synthase. During maturation the amount of mitochondria rises, and, in parallel, citrate synthase gene expression increases. But in failing heart, the mitochondria and citrate synthase are depleted [139].

Adrenergic hyperactivation is associated with high amounts of catecholamines circulating, which promotes reactive oxygen spices (ROS) production. In addition, high amounts of ROS are produced not only by direct stimulation (anthracyclines, tachycardia-induced cardiomyopathy, dilated cardiomyopathy, and etc.) but also by cardiomyocytes overstretch (heart failure with volume overload: valvular diseases, inherited defects) [5, 130, 191].

The main ROS are superoxide ($-O_2$), hydrogen peroxide, and hydroxyl radicals ($-OH$). Increased formation of this compounds promotes lipid membranes perforation of organelles, DNA, and mitochondria injury [202]. Then this leads to a decrease in SR ATPase, Ca^{+2} pump, and Na/K pump and Ca^{+2} accumulation in the cytoplasm [21, 22]. Prolonged exposition to H_2O_2 provokes CA ion oscillations, leading to Ca-dependent protease activation, mitochondrial membranes perforation, and increasing Ca ion flux through mitochondrial membranes. Combinations of these factors provoke myofilament contracture, damage, and petrification of the mitochondria, and proapoptotic factors release [89].

In veterinary literature, there are studies which elucidate some aspects of the antioxidant system and oxidative stress in dogs with the valvular disease. In these studies, an effect of ROS on valvular structures and on pathogenesis was elucidated, but the certain mechanism is still unknown [134, 142].

As described above there are principal differences between healthy and failing hearts; failing hearts have many similarities with fetal heart metabolic profile. The first stages of metabolic adaptation could differ, while the terminal stage of heart failure has a mostly identical phenotype. Unfortunately, myocardial metabolism in veterinary patients with heart failure is not clearly described. We have lack of proper information and can use some information from human medicine studies (mostly on mice and rats and rarely on dogs, cats, ovine, and embryos). Despite new drugs presented on the veterinary pharmacology market, we can treat heart diseases only on clinical stages and do not have pharmacological tools for prophylaxis. Also, we need to provide specific treatment for some inherited forms of myocardial diseases, such as PDK-dependent dilated cardiomyopathy, and identify the role of taurine and carnitine in arrhythmogenic right ventricle dysplasia/cardiomyopathy.

Author details

Dmitrii Oleinikov
Almazov National Medical Research Center, IEM, Research Laboratory of Bioprosthesis and Cardioprotection, Russia

*Address all correspondence to: wolfberg.guard@gmail.com

References

[1] Buchanan CM, Phillips AR, Cooper GJ. Preptin derived from proinsulin-like growth factor II (proIGF-II) is secreted from pancreatic islet beta-cells and enhances insulin secretion. The Biochemical Journal. 2001;**360**:431-439

[2] Cain BS, Meldrum DR, Dinarello CA, Meng X, Banerjee A, Harken AH. Adenosine reduces cardiac TNF-alpha production and human myocardial injury following ischemia-reperfusion. The Journal of Surgical Research. 1998;**76**:117-123

[3] Chandler MP, Kerner J, Huang H, Vazquez E, Reszko A, Martini WZ, et al. Moderate severity heart failure does not involve a downregulation of myocardial fatty acid oxidation. The American Journal of Physiology. 2004;**287**:H1538-H1543

[4] Chen Y, Liu Y, Dorn GW 2nd. Mitochondrial fusion is essential for organelle function and cardiac homeostasis. Circulation Research. 2011;**109**:1327-1331

[5] Cheng W, Kajstura J. Stretch-induced programmed myocyte cell death. The Journal of Clinical Investigation. 1995;**96**:2247-2259

[6] Clark RJ, McDonough PM, Swanson E, Trost SU, Suzuki M, Fukuda M, et al. Diabetes and the accompanying hyperglycemia impairs cardiomyocyte calcium cycling through increased nuclear O-GlcNAcylation. The Journal of Biological Chemistry. 2003;**278**:44230-44237

[7] Clerk A, Bogoyevitch M. Differential activation of protein kinase C isoforms by endothelin-1 and phenylephrine and subsequent stimulation of p42 and p44 mitogen-activated protein kinases in ventricular myocytes cultured from neonatal rat hearts. The Journal of Biological Chemistry. 1994;**269**:32848-32857

[8] Cook G, Edwards T, Jansen M, et al. Differential regulation of carnitine palmitoyltransferase-I gene isoforms (CPT-I alpha and CPT-I beta) in the rat heart. Journal of Molecular and Cellular Cardiology. 2001;**33**:317-329

[9] Cook SA, Varela-Caver A, et al. Abnormal myocardial insulin signaling in type 2 diabetes and left-ventricular dysfunction. European Heart Journal. 2010;**31**:100-111

[10] Cornish J, Callon KE, Bava U, Watson M, Xu X, Lin JM, et al. Preptin, another peptide product of the pancreatic beta-cell, is osteogenic in vitro and in vivo. American Journal of Physiology. Endocrinology and Metabolism. 2007;**292**:E117-E122

[11] Davila-Roman VG, Vedala G, et al. Altered myocardial fatty acid and glucose metabolism in idiopathic dilated cardiomyopathy. Journal of the American College of Cardiology. 2002;**40**(2):271-277

[12] Dawson AG. Oxidation of cytosolic NADH formed during aerobic metabolism in mammalian cells. Trends in Biochemical Sciences. 1979;**4**:171-176

[13] de Lima junior EA, Yamashita AS, et al. Doxorubicin caused severe hyperglycemia and insulin resistance, mediated by inhibition in AMPK in skeletal muscle. Journal of Cachexia, Sarcopenia and Muscle. 2016;**7**(5):615-625

[14] De Meyts P, Roth J, Neville DM Jr, Gavin JR 3rd, Lesniak MA. Insulin interactions with its receptors: Experimental evidence for negative cooperativity. Biochemical and Biophysical Research Communications. 1973;**55**:154-161

[15] De Naeyer H, Ouwens DM, Van Nieuwenhove Y, Pattyn P, 't Hart LM, Kaufman JM, et al. Combined gene and protein expression of hormone-sensitive lipase and adiposetriglyceride lipase, mitochondrial content, and adipocyte size in subcutaneous and visceral adipose tissue of morbidly obese men. Obesity Facts. 2011;**4**:407-416

[16] Dedkova EN, Blatter LA. Mitochondrial Ca2 and the heart. Cell Calcium. 2008;**44**:77-91

[17] Depre C, Hue L. Cyclic GMP in the perfused rat heart. Effect of ischaemia, anoxia and nitric oxide synthase inhibitor. FEBS Letters. 1994;**345**:241-245

[18] Depre C, Gaussin V, Ponchaut S, Fischer Y, Vanoverschelde JL, Hue L. Inhibition of myocardial glucose uptake by cGMP. American Journal of Physiology—Heart and Circulatory Physiology. 1998;**274**:1443-1449

[19] Depre C, Vanoverschelde JL, Goudemant JF, Mottet I, Hue L. Protection against ischemic injury by nonvasoactive concentrations of nitric oxide synthase inhibitors in the perfused rabbit heart. Circulation. 1995;**92**:1911-1918

[20] Des Rosiers C, Labarthe F, Lloyd SG, Chatham JC. Cardiac anaplerosis in health and disease: Food for thought. Cardiovascular Research. 2011;**90**:210-219

[21] Dixon IM, Hata T, Dhalla NS. Sarcolemmal N-K. ATPase activity in congestive heart failure due to myocardial infarction. The American Journal of Physiology. 1992;**262**:C664-C671

[22] Dixon IM, Kaneko M, Hata T, Panagia V, Dhalla NS. Alterations in cardiac membrane Ca transport during oxidative stress. Molecular and Cellular Biochemistry. 1990;**99**:125-133

[23] Doehner W, Rauchhaus M. Impaired insulin sensitivity as an independent risk factor for mortality in patients with stable chronic heart failure. Journal of the American College of Cardiology. 2005;**46**:1019-1026

[24] Doenst T, Pytel G, Schrepper A, Amorim P, Farber G, Shingu Y, et al. Decreased rates of substrate oxidation ex vivo predict the onset of heart failure and contractile dysfunction in rats with pressure overload. Cardiovascular Research. 2010;**86**:461-470

[25] Dorn GW 2nd, Maack C. SR and mitochondria: Calcium cross-talk between kissing cousins. Journal of Molecular and Cellular Cardiology. 2013;**55**:42-49

[26] Dresner A. Effects of free fatty acids on glucose transport and IRS-1-associated phosphatidylinositol 3-kinase activity. The Journal of Clinical Investigation. 1999;**103**:253-259

[27] Dua A, Hennes MI, Hoffmann RG, Maas DL, Krakower GR, Sonnenberg GE, et al. Leptin: A significant indicator of total body fat but not of visceral fat and insulin insensitivity in African-American women. Diabetes. 1996;**45**:1635-1637

[28] Dyck JR, Cheng JF, Stanley WC, Barr R, Chandler MP, Brown S, et al. Malonyl coenzyme a decarboxylase inhibition protects the ischemic heart by inhibiting fatty acid oxidation and stimulating glucose oxidation. Circulation Research. 2004;**94**:78-84

[29] Dzeja PP, Pucar D, Redfield MM, Burnett JC, Terzic A. Reduced activity of enzymes coupling ATP-generating with ATP consuming processes in the failing myocardium. Molecular and Cellular Biochemistry. 1999;**201**:33-40

[30] Fagore S, Chowdhury N. Analyzing methods for path mining with applications in metabolomics. Gene. 2014;**534**:125-138

[31] Fell DA. Increasing the flux in metabolic pathways: A metabolic control analysis perspective. Biotechnology and Bioengineering. 1998;**58**:121-124

[32] Fell DA, Sauro HM. Metabolic control analysis. The effects of high enzyme concentrations. European Journal of Biochemistry. 1990;**192**:183-187

[33] Finck B, Ho Han D, Coleman T. A potential link between muscle PPAR-a signaling and obesity-related diabetes. Cell Metabolism. 2005;**1**:133-144

[34] Fischer Y, Thomas J. Insulin-induced recruitment of GLUT and GLUT1 in isolated rat cardiac myocytes. The Journal of Biological Chemistry, 1997;**272**:7085-7092

[35] Flores NA, Sheridan DJ. Electrophysiological and arrhythmogenic effects of platelet activating factor during normal perfusion myocardial ischemia, and reperfusion in the Guinea pig. British Journal of Pharmacology. 1990;**101**:734-738

[36] Fukushima A, Lopaschuk G. Acetylation control of cardiac fatty acid b-oxidation and energy metabolism in obesity, diabetes and heart failure. Biochimica et Biophysica Acta. 2016;**1862**:2311-3220

[37] Ganesh Kumar K, Zhang J, Gao S, Rossi J, McGuinness OP, Halem HH, et al. Adropin deficiency is associated with increased adiposity and insulin resistance. Obesity (Silver Spring). 2012;**20**:1394-1402

[38] Gao S, McMillan RP, Jacas J, et al. Regulation of substrate oxidation preferences in muscle by the peptide hormone adropin. Diabetes. 2014;**63**(10):3242-3252

[39] Gao S, McMillan RP, Zhu Q, et al. Therapeutic effects of adropin on glucose tolerance and substrate utilization in diet-induced obese mice with insulin resistance. Molecular Metabolism. 2015;**4**(4):310-324

[40] Garcia CK, Goldstein JL, Pathak RK, Anderson RG, Brown MS. Molecular characterization of a membrane transporter for lactate, pyruvate, and other monocarboxylates: Implications for the Cori cycle. Cell. 1994;**76**:865-873

[41] Guillen I, Blanes M, Gomez-Lechon MJ, Castell JV. Cytokine signaling during myocardial infarction: Sequential appearance of IL-1b and IL-6. The American Journal of Physiology. 1995;**269**:R229-R235

[42] Gulick T, Chung MK, Pieper SJ, Lange LG, Schreiner GF. Interleukin-1 and tumor necrosis factor inhibit b-adrenergic responsiveness. Proceedings of the National Academy of Sciences of the United States of America. 1989;**86**:6753-6757

[43] Gurevitch J, Frolkis I, Yuhas Y, et al. Anti-tumor necrosis factor- alpha improves myocardial recovery after ischemia and reperfusion. Journal of the American College of Cardiology. 1997;**30**:1554-1561

[44] Guzun R, Gonzalez-Granillo M, Karu-Varikmaa M, Grichine A, Usson Y, Kaambre T, et al. Regulation of respiration in muscle cells in vivo by VDAC through interaction with the cytoskeleton and MtCK within mitochondrial interactosome. Biochimica et Biophysica Acta. 1818;**2012**:1545-1554

[45] Kim HS, Kang JH. Serum concentrations of leptin and adiponectin in dogs with myxomatous mitral valve disease. Journal of Veterinary Internal Medicine. 2016;**30**:1589-1600

[46] Haemmerle G, Moustafa T, Woelkart G, Buttner S, Schmidt A,

van de Weijer T, et al. ATGL-mediated fat catabolism regulates cardiac mitochondrial function via PPAR-alpha and PGC-1. Nature Medicine. 2011;**17**:1076-1085

[47] Hall JL, Stanley WC, Lopaschuk GD, Wisneski JA, Pizzurro RD, Hamilton CD, et al. Impaired pyruvate oxidation but normal glucose uptake in diabetic pig heart during dobutamine-induced work. American Journal of Physiology—Heart and Circulatory Physiology. 1996;**271**:2320-2329

[48] Hansen P. Role of neutrophils in myocardial ischemia and reperfusion. Circulation. 1995;**91**:1872-1885

[49] Hasselbaink DM, Glatz JF, Luiken JJ, Roemen TH, van der Vusse GJ. Ketone bodies disturb fatty acid handling in isolated cardiomyocytes derived from control and diabetic rats. Biochemical Journal. 2003;**371**:753-760

[50] Hawkins RA: Uptake of ketone bodies by rat brain in vivo. Biochemical Journal. 1971;**121**:17

[51] Hein S, Kostin S, Heling A, et al. The role of the cytoskeleton in heart failure. Cardiovascular Research. 2000;**45**:273-278

[52] Henning S, Wambolt R, Lopaschuk G. Contribution of glycogen to aerobic myocardial glucose metabolism. Circulation. 1996;**93**:1549-1555

[53] Hickson-Bick DL, Buja ML, McMillin JB. Palmitate-mediated alterations in the fatty acid metabolism of rat neonatal cardiac myocytes. Journal of Molecular and Cellular Cardiology. 2000;**32**:511-519

[54] Higgins AJ, Morville M, Burges RA, Gardiner DG, Page MG, Blackburn KJ. Oxfenicine diverts rat muscle metabolism from fatty acid to carbohydrate oxidation and protects the ischaemic rat heart. Life Sciences. 1980;**27**:963-970

[55] Houtkooper RH, Canto C, Wanders RJ, Auwerx J. The secret life of nad: An old metabolite controlling new metabolic signaling pathways. Endocrine Reviews. 2010;**31**:194-223

[56] Hu Y, Belke D, Suarez J, Swanson E, Clark R, Hoshijima M, et al. Adenovirusmediated overexpression of O-GlcNAcase improves contractile function in the diabetic heart. Circulation Research. 2005;**96**:1006-1013

[57] Hue L, Depre C. Regulation of glucose metabolism in cardiac muscle. Biochemical Society Transactions. 1995;**23**:311-314

[58] Huges W, Denton R. Incorporation of 32P1 into PDH phosphatase in mitochondria from control and insulin-treated adipose tissue. Nature. 1976;**264**:471-473

[59] Huss J, Kelly D. Unclear receptor signaling and cardiac energetics. Circulation Research. 2004;**95**:613-623

[60] Ingwall JS. ATP and the Heart. Norwell, MA: Kluwer Academic; 2002

[61] Ingwall JS. Energy metabolism in heart failure and remodelling. Cardiovascular Research. 2009;**81**:412-419

[62] Jastroch M, Divakaruni AS, Mookerjee S, Treberg JR, Brand MD. Mitochondrial proton and electron leaks. Essays in Biochemistry. 2010;**47**:53-67

[63] Jaswal JS, Keung W, Wang W, Ussher JR, Lopaschuk GD. Targeting fatty acid and carbohydrate oxidation—A novel therapeutic intervention in the ischemic and failing heart. Biochimica et Biophysica Acta. 1813;**2011**:1333-1350

[64] Johannsson E, Nagelhus EA, McCullagh KJ, Sejersted OM,

Blackstad TW, Bonen A, et al. Cellular and subcellular expression of the monocarboxylate transporter MCT1 in rat heart. A high-resolution immunogold analysis. Circulation Research. 1997;**80**:400-407

[65] Joubert F, Wilding JR, Fortin D, Domergue-Dupont V, Novotova M, Ventura-Clapier R, et al. Local energetic regulation of sarcoplasmic and myosin ATPase is differently impaired in rats with heart failure. The Journal of Physiology. 2008;**586**:5181-5192

[66] Kaasik A, Veksler V, Boehm E, Novotova M, Minajeva A, Ventura-Clapier R. Energetic crosstalk between organelles: Architectural integration of energy production and utilization. Circulation Research. 2001;**89**:153-159

[67] Kaijser L, Berglund B. Myocardial lactate extraction and release at rest and during heavy exercise in healthy men. Acta Physiologica Scandinavica. 1992;**144**:39-45

[68] Kampf JP, Parmley D, Kleinfeld AM. Free fatty acid transport across adipocytes is mediated by an unknown membrane protein pump. American Journal of Physiology. Endocrinology and Metabolism. 2007;**293**:E1207-E1214

[69] Kanehisa M. KEGG database. Novartis Foundation Symposium. 2002;**547**:91-101

[70] Kelly R, Balligandd JL. Nitric oxide and cardiac function. Circulation Research. 1996;**79**:363-380

[71] Kerbel B, Unniappan S. Nesfatin-1 suppresses energy intake, co-localises ghrelin in the brain and gut, and alters ghrelin, cholecystokinin and orexin mRNA expression in goldfish. Journal of Neuroendocrinology. 2012;**24**:366-377

[72] Kerner J, Hoppel CL. Radiochemical malonyl-CoA decarboxylase assay: Activity and subcellular distribution in heart and skeletal muscle. Analytical Biochemistry. 2002;**306**:283-289

[73] Kim H, Kim D, Lee I, et al. Human fetal heart development after mid-term: Morphometry and ultrastructural study. Journal of Molecular and Cellular Cardiology. 1992;**24**:949-965

[74] Kinugawa K, Takahashi T, Kohmoto O, et al. Nitric oxide-mediated effects of interleukin-6 on [Ca] and cell contraction in cultured chick ventricular myocytes. Circulation Research. 1994;**75**:285-295

[75] Kjekshus JK, Mjos OD. Effect of free fatty acids on myocardial function and metabolism in the ischemic dog heart. Journal of Clinical Investigation. 1972;**51**:1767-1776

[76] Knupfer C, Beckstein C. Structure, function and behavior of computational models in system biology. BMC Systems Biology. 2013;**7**:43

[77] Kojima M, Hosoda H, Date Y, Nakazato M, Matsuo H, Kangawa K. Ghrelin is a growth-hormone-releasing acylated peptide from stomach. Nature. 1999;**402**:656-660

[78] Koonen DP, Glatz JF, Bonen A, Luiken JJ. Long-chain fatty acid uptake and FAT/CD36 translocation in heart and skeletal muscle. Biochimica et Biophysica Acta. 1736;**2005**:163-180

[79] Korvald C, Elvenes OP, Myrmel T. Myocardial substrate metabolism influences left ventricular energetics in vivo. American Journal of Physiology—Heart and Circulatory Physiology. 2000;**278**:1345-1351

[80] Kotoulas OB, Kalamidas SA, Kondomerkos DJ. Glycogen autophagy. Microscopy Research and Technique. 2004;**64**:10-20

[81] Krssak M. Intramyocellular lipid concentrations are correlated with

insulin sensitivity in humans: A 1H NMR spectroscopy study. Diabetologia. 1999;**42**:113-116

[82] Kumar KG, Trevaskis JL, Lam DD, Sutton GM, Koza RA, Chouljenko VN, et al. Identification of adropin as a secreted factor linking dietary macronutrient intake with energy homeostasis and lipid metabolism. Cell Metabolism. 2008;**8**:468-481

[83] Kurzelewski M, Duda M, Stanley WC, Boemke W, Beresewicz A. Nitric oxide synthase inhibition and elevated endothelin increase oxygen consumption but do not affect glucose and palmitate oxidation in the isolated rat heart. Journal of Physiology and Pharmacology. 2004;**55**:27-38

[84] Lanner JT. Ryanodine receptor physiology and its role in disease. Advances in Experimental Medicine and Biology. 2012;**740**:217-234

[85] LaNoue KF, Williamson JR. Interrelationships between malate-aspartate shuttle and citric acid cycle in rat heart mitochondria. Metabolism. 1971;**20**:119-140

[86] Laughlim M, Taylor J. Non-glucose substrates increase glycogen synthesis in vivo in dog heart. The American Journal of Physiology. 1994;**267**:H217-H223

[87] Lehman JJ, Kelly DP. Gene regulatory mechanisms governing energy metabolism during cardiac hypertrophic growth. Heart Failure Reviews. 2002;**7**:175-185

[88] Lester JW, Hofmann PA. Role of PKC in the adenosine-induced decrease in shortening velocity of rat ventricular myocytes. The American Journal of Physiology. 2000;**279**:H2685-H2693

[89] Li C, Jackson R. Reactive species mechanisms of cellular hypoxia-reoxygenation injury. American Journal of Physiology—Cell Physiology. 2002;**282**:227-241

[90] Li O, Zhu X, Ishikura S. Ca^{+2} signals promote GLUT4 exocytosis and reduce its endocytosis in muscle cells. American Journal of Physiology—Endocrinology and Metabolism, 2014;**307**:E209-E224

[91] Lian W, Gu X, Qin Y, Zheng X. Elevated plasma levels of adropin in heart failure patients. Internal Medicine. 2011;**50**:1523-1527

[92] Liao R, Jain M, Cui L, D'Agostino J, Aiello F, Luptak I, et al. Cardiac-specific overexpression of GLUT1 prevents the development of heart failure attributable to pressure overload in mice. Circulation. 2002;**106**:2125-2131

[93] Lin SJ, Guarente L. Nicotinamide adenine dinucleotide, a metabolic regulator of transcription, longevity and disease. Current Opinion in Cell Biology. 2003;**2**:241-246

[94] Lionetti V, Guiducci L, Aquaro GD, et al. Mismatch between uniform increase in cardiac glucose uptake and regional contractile dysfunction in pacing-induced heart failure. American Journal of Physiology: Heart and Circulatory Physiology. 2007;**293**:2747-2756

[95] Little JR, Goto M, Spitzer JJ. Effect of ketones on metabolism of FFA by dog myocardium and skeletal muscle in vivo. American Journal of Physiology. 1970;**219**:1458-1463

[96] Liu J, Wang C, Murakami Y, et al. Mitochondrial ATPase and high-energy phosphates in failing hearts. American Journal of Physiology. Heart and Circulatory Physiology. 2001;**281**:H1319-H1326

[97] Lopaschuk G, Collins-Nakai R, Itoi T. Developmental changes in energy substrate use by the heart. Cardiovascular Research. 1992;**26**:1172-1180

[98] Lopaschuk GD, Ussher JR, Folmes CD, Jaswal JS, Stanley WC. Myocardial fatty acid metabolism in health and disease. Physiological Reviews. 2010;**90**:207-258

[99] Lopaschuk GD, Wall SR, Olley PM, Davies NJ. Etomoxir, a carnitine palmitoyltransferase I inhibitor, protects hearts from fatty acid-induced ischemic injury independent of changes in long chain acylcarnitine. Circulation Research. 1988;**63**:1036-1043

[100] Luiken JJ, Koonen DP, Willems J, Zorzano A, Becker C, Fischer Y, et al. Insulin stimulates long-chain fatty acid utilization by rat cardiac myocytes through cellular redistribution of FAT/CD36. Diabetes. 2002;**51**:3113-3119

[101] Luiken JJ, Schaap FG, van Nieuwenhoven FA, van der Vusse GJ, Bonen A, Glatz JF. Cellular fatty acid transport in heart and skeletal muscle as facilitated by proteins. Lipids. 1999;**34**:S169-S175

[102] Luiken JJ, Willems J, van der Vusse GJ, Glatz JF. Electrostimulation enhances FAT/CD36-mediated long-chain fatty acid uptake by isolated rat cardiac myocytes. American Journal of Physiology—Endocrinology and Metabolism. 2001;**281**:704-712

[103] Lundgrin EL, Park MM, Sharp J, Tang WH, Thomas JD, Asosingh K, et al. Fasting 2-deoxy-2-[18F] fluoro-D-glucose positron emission tomography to detect metabolic changes in pulmonary arterial hypertension hearts over 1 year. Annals of the American Thoracic Society. 2013;**10**:1-9

[104] Massie BM, Schwartz GG, Garcia J, Wisneski JA, Weiner MW, Owens T. Myocardial metabolism during increased work states in the porcine left ventricle in vivo. Circulation Research. 1994;**74**:64-73

[105] Mathias S, Dressler KA, Kolesnik RN. Characterization of a ceramide-activated protein kinase: Stimulation by tumor necrosis alpha. Proceedings of the National Academy of Sciences of the United States of America. 1991;**88**:10009-10013

[106] McCormack JD, Denton RM. Role of Ca^2 ions in the regulation of intramitochondrial metabolism in rat heart. Evidence from studies with isolated mitochondria that adrenaline activates the pyruvate dehydrogenase and 2-oxoglutarate dehydrogenase complexes by increasing the intramitochondrial concentration of Ca^2. Biochemical Journal. 1984;**218**:235-247

[107] McCormack JG, Denton RM. Influence of calcium ions on mammalian intramitochondrial dehydrogenases. Methods in Enzymology. 1989;**174**:95-118

[108] McGarry JD, Dobbins RL. Fatty acids, lipotoxicity and insulin secretion. Diabetologia. 1999;**42**:128-138

[109] Mjos OD, Kjekshus J. Increased local metabolic rate by free fatty acids in the intact dog heart. Scandinavian Journal of Clinical and Laboratory Investigation. 1971;**28**:389-393

[110] Montessuit C, Thorburn A. Transcriptional activation of the glucose transporter GLUT1 in ventricular cardiac myocytes by hypertrophic agonists. The Journal of Biological Chemistry. 1999;**274**:9006-9012

[111] Mootha VK, Arai AE, Balaban RS. Maximum oxidative phosphorylation capacity of the mammalian heart. American Journal of Physiology—Heart and Circulatory Physiology. 1997;**272**:769-775

[112] Mori J, Basu R, McLean BA, Das SK, Zhang L, Patel VB, et al.

Agonist-induced hypertrophy and diastolic dysfunction are associated with selective reduction in glucose oxidation: A metabolic contribution to heart failure with normal ejection fraction. Circulation. Heart Failure. 2012;**5**:493-503

[113] Nakao K, Minobe W, Roden R, et al. Myosin heavy chain gene expression in human heart failure. The Journal of Clinical Investigation. 1997;**100**:2362-2370

[114] Neubauer S, Horn M, Cramer M, Harre K, Newell JB, Peters W, et al. Myocardial phosphocreatine-to-ATP ratio is a predictor of mortality in patients with dilated cardiomyopathy. Circulation. 1997;**96**:2190-2196

[115] Neubauer S. The failing heart—An engine out of fuel. New England Journal of Medicine. 2007;**356**:1140-1151

[116] Nikolaidis LA, Sturzu A, Stolarski C, Elahi D, Shen YT, Shannon RP. The development of myocardial insulin resistance in conscious dogs with advanced dilated cardiomyopathy. Cardiovascular Research. 2004;**61**:297-306

[117] O'Donnell JM, Fields AD, Sorokina N, Lewandowski ED. The absence of endogenous lipid oxidation in early stage heart failure exposes limits in lipid storage and turnover. Journal of Molecular and Cellular Cardiology. 2008;**44**:315-322

[118] O'Donnell JM, White LT, Lewandowski ED. Mitochondrial transporter responsiveness and metabolic flux homeostasis in postischemic hearts. American Journal of Physiology. 1999;**277**:866-873

[119] O'Rourke B, Blatter LA. Mitochondrial Ca^2 uptake: Tortoise or hare? Journal of Molecular and Cellular Cardiology. 2009;**46**:767-774

[120] Oh-I S, Shimizu H, Satoh T, Okada S, Adachi S, Inoue K, et al. Identification of nesfatin-1 as a satiety molecule in the hypothalamus. Nature. 2006;**443**:709-712

[121] Oleynikov D, Vasilieva S, Jashin A. Testosterone and myocardial extract as a correction scheme in case of experimental doxorubicin cardiomyopathy. Canadian Scientific Journal. 2015;**1**:4-10

[122] Opie LH, Thandroyen FT, Muller C, Bricknell OL. Adrenaline-induced "oxygen-wastage" and enzyme release from working rat heart. Effects of calcium antagonism, beta-blockade, nicotinic acid and coronary artery ligation. Journal of Molecular and Cellular Cardiology. 1979;**11**:1073-1094

[123] Oral H, Dorn GW, Mann DL. Sphingosine mediates the immediate negative inotropic effects of tumor necrosis factor-a in the adult mammalian cardiac myocyte. The Journal of Biological Chemistry. 1997;**272**:4836-4842

[124] Osawa H, Robey R, Printz R. Analysis of signaling pathway involved in the regulation of hexokinase 2 gene transcription by insulin. The Journal of Biological Chemistry. 1996;**271**:16690-16694

[125] Ostrander DB, Sparagna GC, Amoscato AA, McMillin JB, Dowhan W. Decreased cardiolipin synthesis corresponds with cytochrome c release in palmitate-induced cardiomyocyte apoptosis. Journal of Biological Chemistry. 2001;**276**:38061-38067

[126] Ozkan Y, Timurkan ES, Aydin S, Sahin I, Timurkan M, Citil C, et al. Acylated and desacylated ghrelin, preptin, leptin, and nesfatin-1 peptide changes related to the body mass index. International Journal of Endocrinology. 2013. 7 pages. Article ID: 236085

[127] Panagia M, Gibbons G, Radda G. PPAR-a activation required for decreased glucose uptake and increased susceptibility to injury during ischemia. American Journal of Physiology. Heart and Circulatory Physiology. 2005;**288**:H2677-H2683

[128] Paolisso G, De Riu S, Marrazzo G, Verza M, Varricchio M, D'Onofrio F. Insulin resistance and hyperinsulinemia in patients with chronic congestive heart failure. Metabolism. 1991;**40**:972-977

[129] Piao L, Fang YH, Cadete VJ, Wietholt C, Urboniene D, Toth PT, et al. The inhibition of pyruvate dehydrogenase kinase improves impaired cardiac function and electrical remodeling in two models of right ventricular hypertrophy: Resuscitating the hibernating right ventricle. Journal of Molecular Medicine. 2010;**88**:47-60

[130] Pimentel D, Amin J. Reactive oxygen species mediate amplitude-dependent hypertrophic and apoptotic responses to mechanical stretch in cardiac myocytes. Circulation Research. 2001;**89**:453-460

[131] Postic C, Leturque A, Printz RL, Maulard P, Loizeau M, Granner DK, et al. Development and regulation of glucose transporter and hexokinase expression in rat. The American Journal of Physiology. 1994;**266**:E548-E559

[132] Postic C, Rencurel F. Girard J. The effects of hyperinsulinemia and hyperglycemia on GLUT4 and hexokinase 2 mRNA and protein in rat skeletal and adipose tissue. Diabetes. 1993;**42**:922-929

[133] Pound KM, Sorokina N, Ballal K, Berkich DA, Fasano M, Lanoue KF, et al. Substrate-enzyme competition attenuates upregulated anaplerotic flux through malic enzyme in hypertrophied rat heart and restores triacylglyceride content: Attenuating upregulated anaplerosis in hypertrophy. Circulation Research. 2009;**104**:805-812

[134] Prasad K, Gupta J. Oxidative stress as a mechanism of cardiac failure in chronic volume overload in canine model. Journal of Molecular and Cellular Cardiology. 1996;**28**:375-385

[135] Ramanjaneya M, Chen J, Brown JE, Tripathi G, Hallschmid M, Patel S, et al. Identification of nesfatin-1 in human and murine adipose tissue: A novel depot-specific adipokine with increased levels in obesity. Endocrinology. 2010;**151**:3169-3178

[136] Randle PJ, Garland PB, Hales CN, Newsholme EA. The glucose fatty-acid cycle: Its role in insulin sensitivity and the metabolic disturbances of diabetes mellitus. Lancet. 1963;**1**:785-789

[137] Randle PJ. Fuel selection in animals. Biochemical Society Transactions. 1986;**14**:799-806

[138] Randle PJ, Priesman DA. Short term and longer term regulation of pyruvate dehydrogenase kinase. In: Alpha-keto Acid Dehydrogenase Complexes. Basel: Birkhauser Verlag; 1996. pp. 151-161

[139] Razeghi P, Young M. Metabolic gene expression in fetal and failing human heart. Circulation. 2001;**11**:2923-2931

[140] Recchia FA, Osorio JC, Chandler MP, Xu X, Panchal AR, Lopaschuk GD, et al. Reduced synthesis of NO causes marked alterations in myocardial substrate metabolism in conscious dogs. American Journal of Physiology—Endocrinology and Metabolism. 2002;**282**:197-206

[141] Rechelt ME, Mellor KM, et al. Myocardial glycophagy—A specific glycogen handling response to metabolic stress is accentuated in the female heart. Journal of Molecular and Cellular cardiology. 2013;**65**:67-75

[142] Reimann M, Haggstrom J. Markers of oxidative stress in dogs with myxomatous mitral valve disease are influenced by sex, neuter status and serum cholesterol concentration. Journal of Veterinary Internal Medicine. 2017;**31**:295-302

[143] Reiser P, Portman M, Ning X, et al. Human cardiac myosin heavy chain isoforms in fetal and failing adult atria and ventricles. The American Journal of Physiology. 2001;**280**:H1814-H1820

[144] Roca-Rivada A, Castelao C, Senin LL, Landrove MO, Baltar J, Belén Crujeiras A, et al. FNDC5/irisin is not only a myokine but also an adipokine. PLoS One. 2013;**8**:e60563

[145] Romano S, Valayannopoulos V, Touati G, Jais JP, Rabier D, de Keyzer Y, et al. Cardiomyopathies in propionic aciduria are reversible after liver transplantation. The Journal of Pediatrics. 2014;**156**:128-134

[146] Rupert BE, Segar JL, Schutte BC, Scholz TD. Metabolic adaptation of the hypertrophied heart: Role of the malate/aspartate and alpha-glycerophosphate shuttles. Journal of Molecular and Cellular Cardiology. 2000;**32**:2287-2297

[147] Ruskoaho H, Lang R, Toth M, et al. Release and regulation of atrial natriuretic peptide (ANP). European Heart Journal. 1987;**8**:99-109

[148] Sabbadini RA, Betto R, Teresi A, Fachechi-Cassano G, Salviati G. The effects of sphingosine on sarcoplasmic reticulum calcium release. The Journal of Biological Chemistry. 1992;**267**:15475-15484

[149] Santalucia T, Camps M, Castello A, et al. Developmental regulation of GLUT-1 (erythroid/HepG2) and GLUT-4 (muscle/fat) glucose transporter expression in rat heart, skeletal muscle, and brown adipose tissue. Endocrinology. 1992;**130**:837-846

[150] Schaffer JE. Lipotoxicity: When tissues overeat. Current Opinion in Lipidology. 2003;**14**:281-287

[151] Unger RH. Lipotoxic diseases. Annual Review of Medicine. 2002;**53**:319-336

[152] Shanik MH, Xu Y, et al. Insulin resistance and hyperinsulinemia. Diabetes Care. 2008;**31**:262-268

[153] Shibayama J, Yuzyuk TN, Cox J, Zaitsev AV, et al. Metabolic remodeling in moderate synchronous versus dyssynchronous pacing-induced heart failure; integrated metabolomics and proteomics study. PLoS One. 2015;**10**(3):32

[154] Simonsen S, Kjekshus JK. The effect of free fatty acids on myocardial oxygen consumption during atrial pacing and catecholamine infusion in man. Circulation. 1978;**58**:484-491

[155] Singh SN, Vats P, Shyam R, Suri S, Kumria MM, Ranganathan S, et al. Role of neuropeptide Y and galanin in high altitude induced anorexia in rats. Nutritional Neuroscience. 2001;**4**:323-331

[156] Solomon SD, St John SM, Lamas GA, Plappert T, Rouleau JL, Skali H, et al. Ventricular remodeling does not accompany the development of heart failure in diabetic patients after myocardial infarction. Circulation. 2002;**106**:1251-1255

[157] Sommerschild HT, Kirkeboen KA. Adenosine and cardioprotection during ischaemia and reperfusion—An overview. Acta Anaesthesiologica Scandinavica. 2000;**44**:1038-1055

[158] Sparagna GC, Hickson-Bick DL, Buja LM, McMillin JB. A metabolic role for mitochondria in palmitate-induced cardiac myocyte apoptosis. American Journal of Physiology—Heart and Circulatory Physiology. 2000;**279**:2124-2132

[159] Stangl V, Baumann G. Negative inotropic mediators released from the heart after myocardial ischaemia-reperfusion. Cardiovascular Research. 2002;**53**:12-30

[160] Stanley WC, Meadows SR, Kivilo KM, Roth BA, Lopaschuk GD. Beta-Hydroxybutyrate inhibits myocardial fatty acid oxidation in vivo independent of changes in malonyl-CoA content. American Journal of Physiology—Heart and Circulatory Physiology. 2003;**285**(4):1626-1631

[161] Stanley WC. Partial fatty acid oxidation inhibitors for stable angina. Expert Opinion on Investigational Drugs. 2002;**11**:615-629

[162] Stanley WC, Lopaschuk GD, McCormack JG. Regulation of energy substrate metabolism in the diabetic heart. Cardiovascular Research. 1997;**34**:25-33

[163] Stanley WC, Connett RJ. Regulation of muscle carbohydrate metabolism during exercise. FASEB Journal. 1991;**5**:2155-2159

[164] Stanley WC, Lopaschuk GD, McCormack JG.. Regulation of myocardial carbohydrate metabolism under normal and ischemic conditions. Potential for pharmacological interventions. Cardiovascular Research. 1997;**33**:243-257

[165] Steinberg H, Brechtel G. Insulin-mediated skeletal muscle vasodilation in nitric oxide-dependent. A novel action of insulate to increase nitric oxide release. The Journal of Clinical Investigation. 1994;**95**:1171-1179

[166] Stengel A, Hofmann T, Goebel-Stengel M, Elbelt U, Kobelt P, Klapp BF. Circulating levels of irisin in patients with anorexia nervosa and different stages of obesity—Correlation with body mass index. Peptides. 2013;**39**:125-130

[167] Stockli J, Fazakerley D, James D. GLUT4 exocytosis. Journal of Cell Science. 2011;**124**:4147-4159

[168] St-Onge MP, Shechter A, Shlisky J, Tam CS, Gao S, Ravussin E, et al. Fasting plasma adropin concentrations correlate with fat consumption in human females. Obesity. Silver Spring; 2014;**22**(4):1056-1063

[169] Swan JW, Anker SD, Walton C, Godsland IF, Clark AL, Leyva F, et al. Insulin resistance in chronic heart failure: Relation to severity and etiology of heart failure. Journal of the American College of Cardiology. 1997;**30**:527-532

[170] Tada H, Thompson CI, Recchia FA, Loke KE, Ochoa M, Smith CJ, et al. Myocardial glucose uptake is regulated by nitric oxide via endothelial nitric oxide synthase in Langendorff mouse heart. Circulation Research. 2000;**86**:270-274

[171] Taegetmeyer H, Young M, Lopaschuk G. Assessing cardiac metabolism. A scientific statement from the American heart association. Circulation Research. 2016;**118**:1659-1701

[172] Taegtmeyer H, Overturf ML. Effects of moderate hypertension on cardiac function and metabolism in the rabbit. Hypertension. 1988;**11**:416-426

[173] Taegtmeyer H. Energy metabolism of the heart: From basic concepts to clinical applications. Current Problems in Cardiology. 1994;**19**:59-113

[174] Takeishi Y, Ping P. Transgenic overexpression of constitutively active protein kinase C causes concentric cardiac hypertrophy. Circulation Research. 2000;**86**:1218-1223

[175] Taylor M, Wallhaus TR, et al. An evaluation of myocardial fatty acid and glucose uptake using PET with [18F]

Fluoro-6-thia-heptadecanoic acid and [18F]FDG in patients with congestive heart failure. The Journal of Nuclear Medicine. 2001;**42**(1):55-62

[176] Tian R, Nascimben L, Kaddurah-Daouk R, Ingwall JS. Depletion of energy reserve via the creatine kinase reaction during the evolution of heart failure in cardiomyopathic hamsters. Journal of Molecular and Cellular Cardiology. 1996;**28**:755-765

[177] Tian R, Abel E. Responses of GLUT4-deficient hearts to ischemia underscore the importance of glycolysis. Circulation. 2001;**103**:2961-2966

[178] Tschöp M, Smiley DL, Heiman ML. Ghrelin induces adiposity in rodents. Nature. 2000;**407**:908-913

[179] Tsujino M, Hirata Y, Imai T, Kanno K, Eguchi S, Hiroshi I. Marumo induction of nitric oxide synthase gene by interleukin-1b in cultured rat cardiocytes. Circulation. 1994;**90**:375-383

[180] Unger RH. Minireview: Weapons of lean body mass destruction: The role of ectopic lipids in the metabolic syndrome. Endocrinology. 2003;**144**:5159-5165

[181] Van der Vusse GJ, van Bilsen M, Glatz JF. Cardiac fatty acid uptake and transport in health and disease. Cardiovascular Research. 2000;**45**:279-293

[182] Veksler V, Ventura-Clapier R. In situ study of myofibrils, mitochondria and bound creatine kinases in experimental cardiomyopathies. Molecular and Cellular Biochemistry. 1994;**133**:287-298

[183] Vendelin M, Beraud N, Guerrero K, Andrienko T, Kuznetsov AV, Olivares J, et al. Mitochondrial regular arrangement in muscle cells: A "crystal-like" pattern. American Journal of Physiology—Cell Physiology. 2005;**288**:C757-C767

[184] Ventura-Clapier R, Garnier A, Veksler V. Energy metabolism in heart failure. The Journal of Physiology. 2004;**555**:1-13

[185] Wakasaki H, Koya D. Targeted overexpression of protein kinase C beta2 isoform in myocardium causes cardiomyopathy. Proceedings of the National Academy of Sciences of the United States of America. 1997;**94**:9320-9325

[186] Wallis M. New insulin-like growth factor (IGF)-precursor sequences from mammalian genomes: The molecular evolution of IGFs and associated peptides in primates. Growth Hormone & IGF Research. 2009;**19**:12-23

[187] Walsh R. The role of angiotensin II in stretch activated signal transduction of the normal, hypertrophied and failing adult heart. In: Dhalla N, Zahradka P. Angiotensin II Blockade: Physiology and Clinical Implications. Boston, Mass: Kluwer Academic Publishers; 1998. pp. 423-434

[188] Ware B, Bevier M, Nishijima Y. Chronic heart failure selectively induces regional heterogeneity of insulin-responsive glucose transporters. American Journal of Physiology. Regulatory, Integrative and Comparative Physiology. 2011;**301**:R1300-R1306

[189] Wilson MA, Cascarano J. The energy-yielding oxidation of nadh by fumarate in submitochondrial particles of rat tissues. Biochimica et Biophysica Acta. 1970;**216**:54-62

[190] Witteles RM, Tang WHW, Jamali AH, et al. Insulin resistance in idiopathic dilated cardiomyopathy. Journal of the American College of Cardiology. 2004;**44**(1):78-81

[191] Wolin MS, Belloni FL. Superoxid anion selectively attenuates catecholamine induced contractile tension in isolated rabbit aorta. The American Journal of Physiology. 1985;**249**:H1227-H1233

[192] Wu ML, Chan CC, Su MJ. Possible mechanism(s) of arachidonic acid-induced intracellular acidosis in rat cardiac myocytes. Circulation Research. 2000;**86**:e55-e62

[193] Wyss M, Smeitnik J. Mitochondrial creatine kinase- a key enzyme of aerobic energy metabolism. Biochimica et Biophysica Acta. 1992;**1102**:119-166

[194] Yagyu H, Chen G, Yokoyama M, Hirata K, Augustus A, Kako Y, et al. Lipoprotein lipase (LpL) on the surface of cardiomyocytes increases lipid uptake and produces a cardiomyopathy. Journal of Clinical Investigation. 2003;**111**:419-426

[195] Yokoyama M, Yagyu H, Hu Y, Seo T, Hirata K, Homma S, et al. Apolipoprotein B production reduces lipotoxic cardiomyopathy: Studies in heart specific lipoprotein lipase transgenic mouse. Journal of Biological Chemistry. 2004;**279**:4204-4211

[196] Young L, Renfu Y. Low-flow ischemia leads to translocation of canine heart GLUT4 and GLUT1 glucose transporter to the sarcolemma in vivo. Circulation. 1997;**95**:415-422

[197] Young ME, Radda GK, Leighton B. Nitric oxide stimulates glucose transport and metabolism in rat skeletal muscle in vitro. Biochemical Journal. 1997;**322**:223-228

[198] Zhang Y, Li R, Meng Y, Li S, Donelan W, Zhao Y, et al. Irisin stimulates browning of white adipocytes through mitogen-activated protein kinase p38 MAP kinase and ERK MAP kinase signaling. Diabetes. 2014;**63**:514-525

[199] Zhang Y, Proenca R, Maffei M, Barone M, Leopold L, Friedman JM. Positional cloning of the mouse obese gene and its human homologue. Nature. 1994;**372**:425-432

[200] Zima A, Pabbidi M, Lipsius S. Effects of mitochondrial uncoupling on Ca^{+2} signaling during excitation-contraction coupling in atrial myocytes. American Journal of Physiology—Heart and Circulatory Physiology. 2013;**304**:H983-H993

[201] Zucker IH. Novel mechanisms of sympathetic regulation in chronic heart failure. Hypertension. 2006;**48**:1005-1011

[202] Zweier JL, Flaherty JT, Weisfeldt ML. Direct measurement of free radical generation following reperfusion of ischemic myocardium. Proceedings of the National Academy of Sciences of the United States of America. 1987;**84**:1404-1407

[203] Hermann G, Dechred GM. The chemical nature of heart failure. Annals of Internal Medicine. 1939;**12**:1233-1244

Chapter 5

Anatomy, Histology, and Physiology of the Canine Prostate Gland

Antonio Fernando Leis-Filho and Carlos E. Fonseca-Alves

Abstract

The prostate gland is the only male accessory gland in dogs and is responsible for secreting the prostatic fluid. Morphologically, the canine prostate gland lacks differentiation into zones, presenting a uniform parenchyma along the longitudinal axis. The luminal epithelial cells secrete a liquid rich in calcium, citric acid, simple sugars, and different enzymes as a component of the seminal plasma. Since the prostatic diseases are very common in small animal practice, there are many information regarding mechanisms of the different prostatic conditions and lack of information regarding the anatomy, histology, and physiology of the canine prostate gland. Thus, this chapter aims to meticulously describe the anatomy, histology, and physiology of the canine prostate gland.

Keywords: dog, prostatic fluid, prostatic tissue, secretory cells, urogenital system

1. Introduction

The prostate gland is the only male accessory gland in dogs, having an important role in the secretion of seminal plasma components. It is a bilobed, oval gland located in the pelvic cavity of adult dogs through which passes the urethra and the vas deferens, where the sperm are carried to the urethra. The prostate communicates with the urethra through several openings along the entire prostatic urethra through which the seminal plasma is secreted. Prostate diseases are extremely common in dogs, so their study is of great importance to better understand these conditions [1, 2]. The castration status is very important for the development of different prostatic disorders [3]. Usually, in developed countries, such as Canada, the United States, and Australia, the castration is very common. Due to castration and low levels of androgen hormones, the prostatic epithelium can be atrophic [1, 2]. On the other hand, the South America countries do not castrate dogs. Then, prostatic disorders such as benign prostatic hyperplasia (BPH) and prostatitis have high incidence [4]. Thus, the knowledge of the anatomy, histology, physiology, and pathology of the canine prostate gland is essential for the better approach of the canine patients.

2. Prostate gland anatomy

The prostate is a semioval bilobular exocrine gland that makes dorsal contact with the rectum, ventral with the pubic symphysis, lateral with the abdominal wall, and cranial with the bladder; its position may present slight variations depending on the age of the dog. Up to 2 months of age, the prostate is located in the caudal portion of the abdominal cavity; from this age until the animal reaches sexual maturity, the prostate is located in the pelvic cavity. After sexual maturity is reached, it increases in size cranially extending into the abdominal cavity [1, 2].

The sulcus dividing the right and left prostate lobes can be palpated dorsally by rectal palpation. Each lobe is subdivided into lobules by trabeculae; these are being formed by composed tubuloalveolar glands, and the ducts of these glands flow into the urethra throughout all its circumference. The prostatic urethra (part of the pelvic urethra that passes through the prostate) crosses the prostatic parenchyma slightly dorsally to its center. In addition, the prostate is covered by a fibromuscular tissue capsule, the prostate capsule [1, 2]. The vas deferens enters the prostate through the cranio-dorsal surface, and each one in a lobe traverses its parenchyma making a caudoventral path ending up in the urethra by the *colliculus seminalis* [1, 2].

The vascularization of the prostate is mainly due to the prostatic artery that originates from the internal pudendal artery. The prostatic artery gives rise to the middle rectal artery that branches and penetrates the prostatic capsule through the dorsolateral surface, becoming subcapsular vessels, until later they enter the prostate to provide the necessary blood supply to the glandular tissue. Anastomoses occur between the prostatic vessels and the urethral, cranial rectal, and caudal arteries, complicating prostatectomy [1, 2].

A venous blood is drained from the prostate by the prostatic and urethral veins to the internal iliac vein. The prostatic lymph vessels drain into the iliac lymph nodes. Prostatic innervation occurs through the hypogastric nerve (sympathetic system), which presents a path similar to the prostatic artery and the pelvic nerve (parasympathetic system). Glandular secretion is increased by parasympathetic stimuli [1, 2].

3. Prostate gland histology

The canine prostate is a morphologically homogeneous organ that does not differentiate into areas such as the human prostate and is mostly composed of secretory glandular tissue (**Figure 1**). The prostatic stroma that surrounds the prostatic urethra extends dorsally and ventrally to almost the limit of the prostate, whereas the lateral projections of the stroma are thinner. These stromal projections subdivide the prostate into several lobules of glandular epithelium. This epithelium is mostly columnar that modifies to cuboid within the ductal structures of

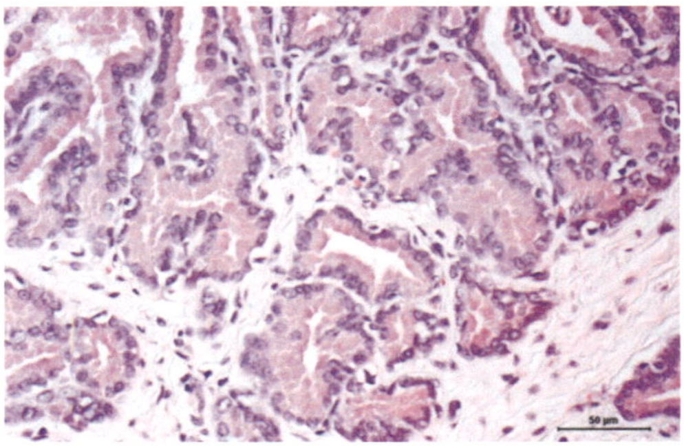

Figure 1.
Canine normal prostate gland. Histological evaluation revealing a columnar epithelium distributed in one layer. The tissue stroma is composed by collagen fibers and fibroblasts. Hematoxylin and eosin (H&E) staining, 10×.

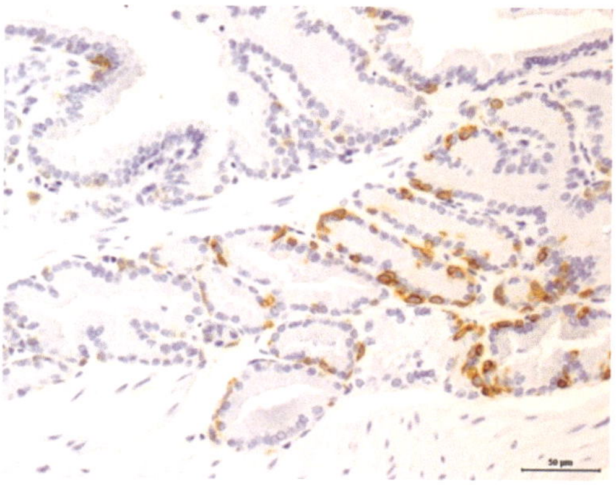

Figure 2.
Immunohistochemical evaluation of high molecular weight cytokeratin (HMWC) in a canine normal prostate gland. It is possible to identify positive membranous staining (brown color) in the basal cells, forming a discontinuous basal cell layer. The luminal cells are negative for the HMWC (blue staining). Harris hematoxylin counterstaining, 3 3'-diaminobenzidine tetrahydrochloride (DAB), 10×.

the prostate; meanwhile the epithelium of the prostatic urethra may be cuboid or columnar, simple, or stratified [5].

The prostatic urethra passes through the prostate gland, showing an urothelial (transitional) epithelium, and the prostatic ducts have connection with the prostatic urethra. Then, inflammatory cells infiltrating the prostatic stroma are common due to the constant antigenic stimulus related with ascended bacteria contamination of the urinary system. Thus, the prostatic stroma is composed by collagen fibers, fibroblast, smooth muscle (for prostatic contraction), and few mononuclear inflammatory cells. In dogs, the smooth muscle cells and the nerves are located in the peripheral region of this gland.

The basal or reserve cells are located in the basal cell layer in a discontinuous distribution (**Figure 2**). Usually, the luminal epithelial cells are positive for cytokeratin 8/18, pan-cytokeratin, NKX3.1, PTEN, and AR [3]. On the other hand, basal cells are positive for cytokeratin 5, p63, and high molecular weight cytokeratins (HMWC) [3].

4. Prostate gland physiology

The prostate is responsible for the production of most of the seminal plasma, which contains large amounts of proteins. One of the most studied proteins in humans, produced by both human and canine prostatic epithelia, is prostate-specific antigen (PSA) [6]. The kallikrein-3 (KLK 3) gene encodes the PSA protein in humans, and dog genome lacks KLK 3 gene. In dogs, kallikrein-2 (canine prostate-specific arginine esterase, (CPSE) is a PSA homolog enzyme belonging to the serine-protease class [6]. This protein is normally secreted into the lumen of the prostate ducts and does not come into contact with the bloodstream in a prostate under physiological conditions. However, when there is a lesion that disrupts the prostate architecture, this protein can be found in the blood and may be an indicator of a prostatic disease [7, 8].

Comparably to PSA, the canine prostate-specific arginine esterase (CPSE) is the most produced protein in the canine prostate and seems to be an alternative for the diagnosis of some prostatic conditions in dogs. Although the use of plasmatic markers as a diagnostic method for prostatic pathologies in human medicine is a commonplace in veterinary medicine, it is not a reality [7, 8].

The prostate depends on the testosterone that is produced in the testicles and converted into dihydrotestosterone (DHT) by the enzyme 5α-reductase. It is known that without this hormonal stimulus, the prostate will decrease its secretory function and volume. Castrated dogs lack testosterone, and consequently DHT will lead the prostate to a state of atrophy [7]. Thus, the endocrine control of the prostate gland, mainly by testis, is well characterized. In male dogs, the testosterone is the most important circulating androgen, and CYP19 (aromatase) can be metabolized into an estradiol-17β. The estrogen can affect the prostate gland growth and differentiation. The role of androgen in prostatic development and pathological process is an understudied area.

5. Prostate gland disorders

5.1 Benign prostatic hyperplasia

Benign prostatic hyperplasia (BPH) is the most common prostatic pathology in dogs. There is a discordance among pathologists regarding the term "BPH." Since hyperplasia is a term applied for a benign growth, using "benign" prostatic "hyperplasia" seems redundant. However, the term BPH is widely accepted in the international literature. Prostatic hyperplasia (PH) or BPH begins as a process of glandular hyperplasia that can occur around the age of 2–3 years. In intact dogs over 9 years, it affects more than 95% of the population [10]. This condition is part of the normal aging process and may include both hyperplastic and hypertrophic processes [1]. Histologically, the PH can be divided into two entities: glandular and complex hyperplasia.

PH is closely related to hormone stimulation in the prostate, indirectly by estrogen and directly by DHT, the former of which causes an increase in the receptors for DHT, and DHT is directly responsible for prostatic growth when binding to epithelial cell receptors of the prostatic cells. In addition, older dogs can present high levels of testosterone production by the testicle that will be converted into DHT in the prostate [1, 9].

Many dogs affected by PH do not show clinical signs until the prostate is large enough to disrupt fecal flow through rectum compression. The most common clinical signs for PH are hematuria, constipation, blood-stained urethral discharge, and hemospermia [10]. The presumptive diagnosis of PH is usually performed by associating the patient's clinical signs with the ultrasonography findings; however, for a definitive diagnosis, the histopathological examination of a prostatic sample is required [1]. The use of ultrasonography is indicated to aid in the evaluation of the extent of the lesion in which the prostate may present as a honeycomb due to the appearance of multiple cysts or as a symmetrical hyperplasia of the gland, which may or may not contain cysts [1, 10].

Neutering is still the most effective and recommended method of treatment of PH in most dogs with a 50–70% decrease in prostate volume at 3 weeks after the surgical procedure; however, the complete decrease of the prostate can take a month [10]. Surgery is contraindicated in cases where the risk of the procedure is too high or if the animal is used for reproduction. In these cases the drug treatment is indicated.

The most commonly used drug for the treatment of PH is finasteride, an inhibitor of 5α-reductase, the enzyme responsible for the conversion of testosterone to DHT. This drug has been widely used in humans for more than 10 years. The use of finasteride decreases prostate volume by 43% after 16 weeks. Although the volume of the ejaculate decreases, the use of finasteride does not alter the seminal quality of the dogs or the libido and may be an option for breeding animals [11].

There are other drugs that may be used as other options for the treatment of PH, such as progestogens, estrogens, analogues, and antagonists of GnRH, but they all have disadvantages when compared to finasteride, either concerning safety of the continuous use of the drug or cost of the drug [1].

5.2 Prostatic cysts

The appearance of prostatic cysts most often is related to PH. Cysts can be classified as intraprostatic or paraprostatic. Intraprostatic or retention cysts arise due to the clogging of the prostatic gland ducts, causing the prostatic fluid to accumulate [9]. At the beginning of this condition, the cysts are very small and not detectable by ultrasonography or rectal palpation, but with the evolution of the condition, many small cysts begin to communicate forming a large cavity that can be detected macroscopically [10, 12].

Paraprostatic cysts are closely associated with remnants of the uterus masculinus, tend to be larger than intraprostatic ones, and can be palpated rectally or even transabdominally [1]. The clinical signs caused by prostatic cysts are very similar to the signs of conditions that cause an increase in prostatic volume, that is, they are reflex of the prostate pressing other structures that are located in the pelvis [12].

The diagnosis of prostatic cysts is performed by ultrasonography, but in cases where the cysts are very small, they may not be detected. The traditional treatment for prostatic cysts is surgical, by any of these techniques: surgical debridement, omentalization, marsupialization, placement of surgical drains, or partial prostatectomy [10, 13, 14].

However, due to the risks of a surgical intervention, new techniques of ultrasound guided drainage are presented as viable options for the treatment of this affection [14].

5.3 Squamous metaplasia

Continuous stimulation of prostatic epithelial cells by estrogen may lead to squamous metaplasia. This estrogenic stimulus may be exogenous or endogenous [15]. The source of endogenous estrogen in animals with squamous metaplasia is the Sertoli cell neoplasia. As in PH, there is a trend toward the formation of prostatic cysts [10].

Squamous metaplasia (**Figure 3**) does not directly cause any clinical signs. This prostatic alteration is reversible if the endogenous or exogenous estrogen source is withdrawn [10].

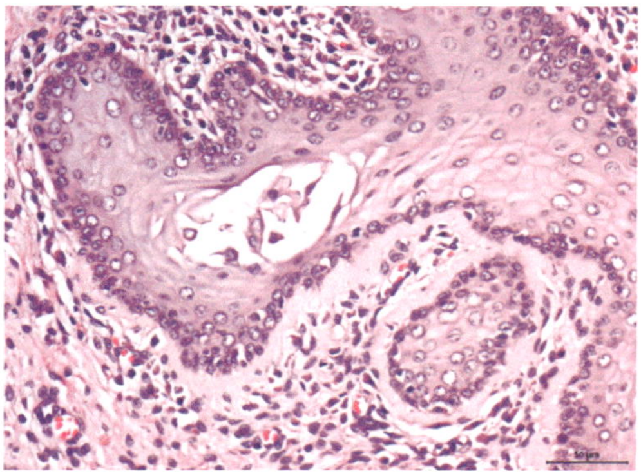

Figure 3.
Canine squamous metaplasia of the prostate gland. It is possible to observe a squamous differentiation of the prostatic epithelium, forming filaments of keratins in the lumen. An inflammatory infiltrate, composed by mononuclear cells, is also observed. Hematoxylin and eosin (H&E) staining, 20×.

5.4 Prostatitis

Prostatitis is a prostate infection that affects mainly older dogs. The origin of the infection can be both ascending by the urinary tract and by hematogenous spread, the second case being rare. Other prostatic conditions such as PH or cysts may compromise the natural defense mechanisms of the prostate and may lead to the development of prostatitis [1, 10].

The most relevant microorganisms linked to prostatitis are *Escherichia coli*, *Staphylococcus*, *Streptococcus* spp., *Mycoplasma* spp., *Proteus*, *Klebsiella* spp., *Pseudomonas aeruginosa*, *Enterobacter*, *Pasteurella* spp., and *Brucella canis*. In rare cases, prostatitis can be caused by fungi [10, 12].

Prostatitis can be divided into two types: acute, in which the infection is more recent and the inflammatory process is more exacerbated and chronic, in which the clinical signs are milder.

The treatment of prostatitis should take into account some key factors for it to be successful. It is of extreme importance for the choice of the drug to evaluate the result of the culture of the prostatic fluid or semen; in addition, one should take into account the pharmacodynamics of the chosen active principle, since the prostate is a tissue of difficult penetration of the antibiotics due to the difference in pH between the prostate fluid and blood [1, 9].

Antibiotic treatment in the case of bacterial prostatitis should last for at least 4 weeks, and a new culture of prostatic fluid and urine should be performed before the end of treatment so that it can be decided between completion and continuation. A new culture test is also recommended 30 days after the end of treatment so that its success is confirmed [1].

Trimethoprim sulfa, chloramphenicol, and enrofloxacin are antibiotics that have good penetration into the prostatic tissue and are therefore good candidates for the treatment of bacterial prostatitis [16].

Castration is indicated as adjuvant therapy to reduce prostate volume and prevent relapse; however, castration should not be performed during acute infection to avoid complications [16].

5.4.1 Acute prostatitis

In acute prostatitis, the infection is more recent, the inflammation is more intense, and the clinical signs presented are anorexia, fever, apathy, vomit, hypogastric region pain, and preputial discharge. In addition, the complete blood count is a characteristic of an acute infectious process, with neutrophilia and left-sided deviation [1].

Diagnosis should be made based on the animal's history and physical examination associated with exams such as transrectal prostate palpation, ultrasonography, complete blood count, urinalysis, and culture of prostate fluid or semen in cases where collection is possible [1].

In prostate palpation, it is common for the animal to present painful sensitivity due to the inflammatory process present there. In ultrasonography, the prostate will most often be enlarged, with its echogenicity increased, and may or may not have associated cysts or abscesses. Urine and semen will most often have neutrophils and bacteria present [1].

5.4.2 Chronic prostatitis

Unlike acute prostatitis, few chronic or no clinical signs are exhibited by the animal. The most common are recurrent urinary tract infections and bloody urethral discharge. In addition, in rectal palpation, the prostate often has a normal volume, and the animal has no painful sensitivity. Because of this, the diagnosis in this case is more difficult and should be based on the clinical findings associated with ultrasonography and culture of the prostatic fluid or semen [1, 9].

The difference of "acute" and "chronic" is usually a clinical classification, since both entities present a very divergent clinical signs, prognosis, and treatment. In a pathological "view," inflammation is usually classified into focal or multifocal and according to the inflammatory infiltrate (cell type involved) and the presence or absence of intraluminal infiltration.

In humans, the chronic inflammatory infiltrate associated with the epithelial atrophy is described as a proliferative inflammatory atrophy (PIA) and is considered as a preneoplastic lesion [17]. In dogs, PIA is also found (**Figure 4**).

5.5 Prostatic abscesses

Prostatic abscesses can be consequences of prostatic cysts that become contaminated or of prostatitis. In the case of prostatitis, tissue inflammation can induce obstruction of the prostatic ducts, causing contaminated contents to accumulate resulting in an abscess [18].

The diagnosis is achieved through the association of history, clinical signs, and complementary tests. The signs of prostatic abscesses are related to the increased prostatic volume, the most common being tenesmus and dysuria. In addition, the animal may or may not feel pain during rectal palpation of the prostate. Ultrasonography and culture of the prostatic fluid are important tests for the diagnosis of prostatic abscesses [1, 14].

The treatment is based on draining the contents of the abscess. The most traditional ones are surgical intervention such as debridement and omentalization, marsupialization, subtotal prostatectomy, or placement of multiple penrose drains. However, due to the risks associated with these procedures, new approaches are emerging [14].

An alternative to the traditional surgical approach is the percutaneous drainage of the abscesses guided by ultrasonography, which in addition to being a cheaper technique than traditional surgery proved to be safe and effective. In addition, antibiotic therapy based on the result of prostatic fluid culture should be instituted in association with the technique chosen for drainage of the abscess [14].

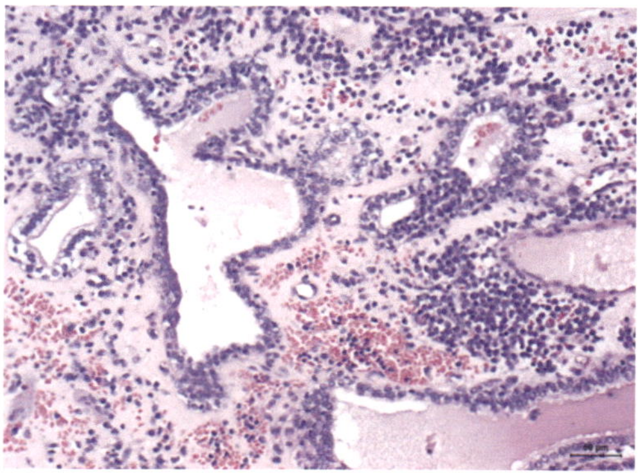

Figure 4.
Canine prostatic atrophic epithelium. There is atrophy of the glandular epithelium, disposed in two or more layers. There is an intense inflammatory mononuclear infiltrate and hemorrhage. Hematoxylin and eosin (H&E) staining, 10×.

5.6 Prostatic neoplasia

Prostatic adenocarcinomas are a rare condition, affecting both castrated and non-castrated animals. They present a prevalence of 0.2–0.6% and have a predilection for animals with more advanced age, and the average age of an animal diagnosed with prostatic neoplasia is around 10 years [19]. Castrated dogs may present a greater chance of developing prostatic adenocarcinoma, being up to 2.38 times greater than non-castrated dogs [19]. In addition, prostatic carcinoma in dogs is androgen independent so castration is not a therapeutic possibility, except in cases associated with PH [16].

In the author's experience, intact dogs present a higher prevalence of prostate cancer (PC), and this can be related to our dog population. Usually, castration is not performed in male dogs. Thus, we have a majority population of intact dogs. In a previous study of our research group [20], we have described a tumor phenotype in 90 canines with PC, and all dogs (90/90) were intact. We did not find any PC in a castrated dog, probably because in our dog population, castration is not routinely performed.

The clinical signs associated with prostatic carcinoma are dysuria, tenesmus, hematuria, anorexia, and weight loss. In addition, through transrectal palpation, the prostate is most often enlarged and asymmetric, and the animal may or may not present pain [16]. Complementary tests such as ultrasound and X-ray should always be required to assess the extent of the neoplasm in both the prostate and possible metastasis. Common radiographic findings are prostatic enlargement, prostatic mineralization, sublumbar lymphadenopathy, axial skeletal metastasis, pulmonary metastasis, and appendicular skeletal metastasis [19].

In ultrasonography, the most common findings are prostatic enlargement, prostatic tissue mineralization, diffuse areas presenting hyperechogenicity, and irregular prostatic contour [19]. Areas of metastasis of prostatic carcinoma in descending order of incidence include the lungs, regional lymph nodes, liver, urethra, spleen, colon, rectum, urinary bladder, bones, heart, liver, and distal and adrenal lymph nodes [16].

The definitive diagnosis of prostatic carcinoma is made by means of cytology or prostate biopsy. Both techniques can be performed transabdominally with the aid of ultrasonography. There are different histological subtypes of prostatic adenocarcinoma, and the major challenge is the differentiation between urothelial and luminal origins of the undifferentiated subtypes. The castrated dogs are more prone to develop the most undifferentiated kinds of neoplasms and seem difficult

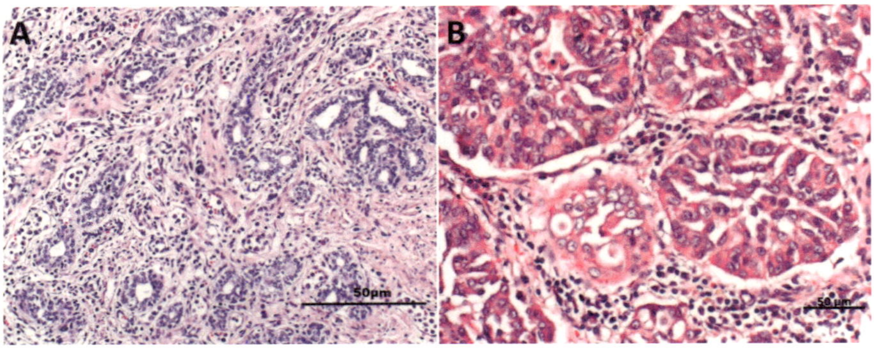

Figure 5.
Canine prostate cancer. (A) Low-grade canine prostate cancer (Gleason score 6) composed by small glandular proliferation with tubules showing more than two layers with evident nucleoli. Hematoxylin and eosin (H&E) staining, 10×. (B) High-grade prostate cancer (Gleason score 8), showing moderate anisokaryosis, evident nucleoli, and mitosis. Hematoxylin and eosin (H&E) staining, 40×.

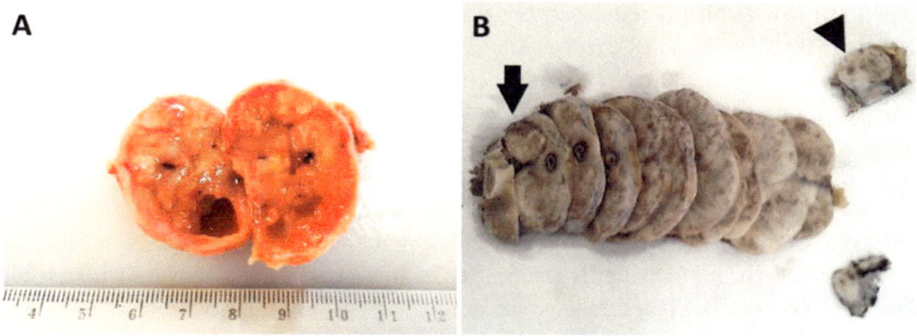

Figure 6.
Gross morphology of two canine prostate cancers. (A) Infiltrative prostate cancer, with the prostate gland showing a heterogeneous parenchyma, cystic areas, and necrosis. (B) A serial section of a prostate gland with a canine prostate cancer showing a well-delimited mass (arrows).

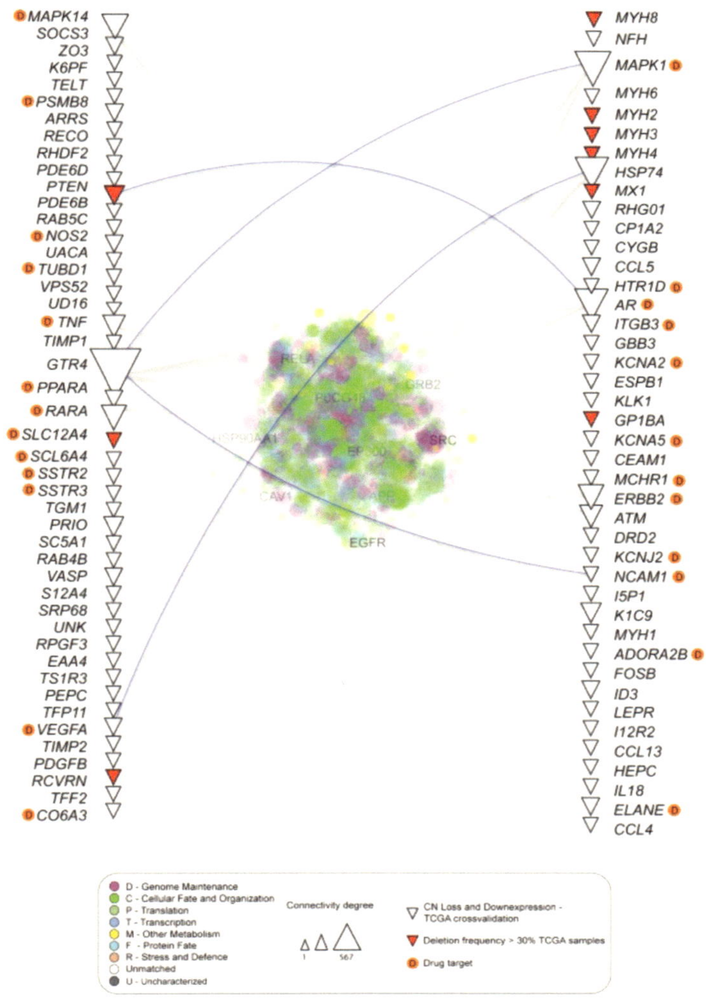

Figure 7.
Protein-protein interaction (PPI) analysis using the canine data (copy number alteration provided by Amorim et al. [27]) and the human prostate cancer data from The Cancer Genome Atlas (TCGA). It is possible to evaluate the connectivity degree between gene alterations in human and dogs (triangles). Genes with deletion frequency higher than 30% (red triangles) and genes with developed drug targets are also observed.

to differentiate an undifferentiated prostatic adenocarcinoma from an undifferentiated prostatic urothelial carcinoma [21]. Recently, the Gleason score was also proposed in canine prostatic pathology (**Figure 5**) [22].

Morphologically, canine PC can present an infiltrative growth pattern or form a prostatic mass (**Figure 6**). The infiltrative pattern can be difficult to differentiate from other prostatic diseases such as prostatitis and PH. Thus, in these cases, ultrasound examination can be challenging.

The treatment of prostatic adenocarcinoma is most often ineffective, making it palliative rather than curative. In addition, in most cases the diagnosis is made only at an advanced stage of the disease, making the prognosis even more reserved [1]. The results of chemotherapy and surgical protocols in cases of prostatic adenocarcinoma are unsatisfactory, not prolonging the life expectancy of the patient. Radiotherapy may be an option in cases where increased prostatic volume due to the tumoral mass is a problem for the animal, since this therapeutic option can cause reduction of the prostate volume but without increase in life expectancy [8].

Another important point to consider is if the animal is neutered or not. Castration or the use of finasteride may help in reducing the prostatic volume but

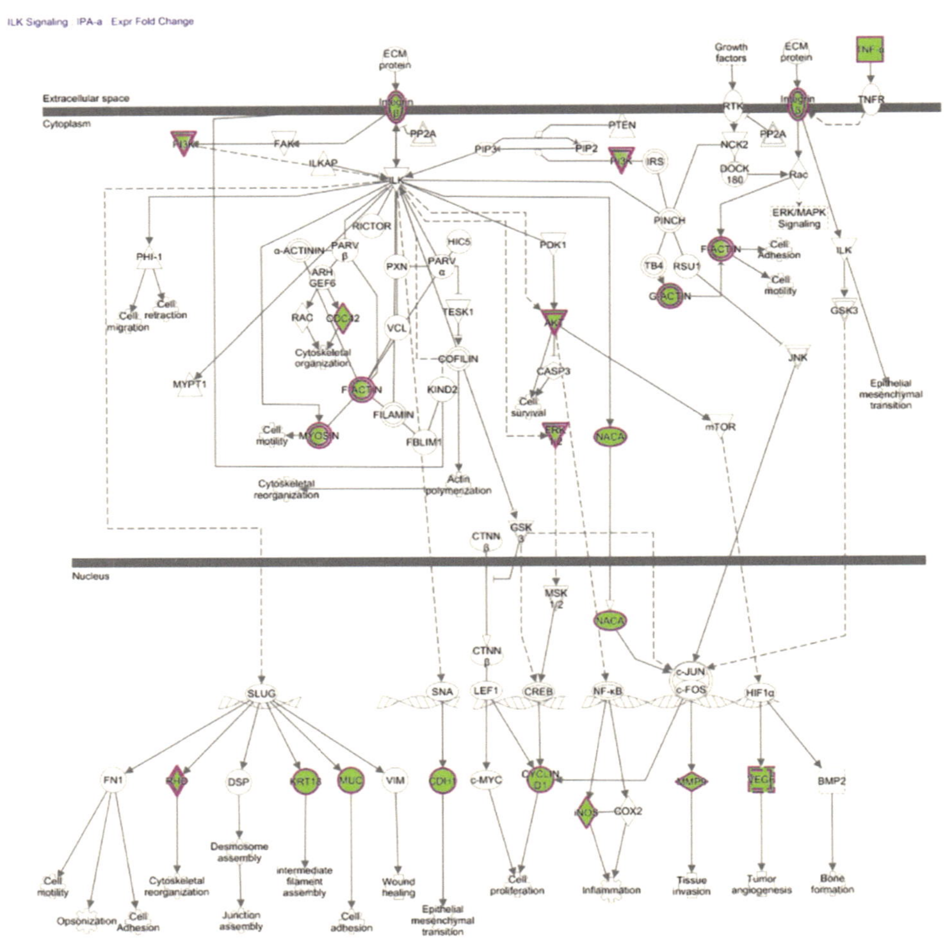

Figure 8.
Ingenuity pathway analysis (IPA) of the canine copy number alteration data published by Amorim et al. [27]. Disruption of the ILK signaling pathway. Genes in green present a significant copy number loss compared to normal tissue.

without influence on the tumor mass. Due to the poor prognosis of this condition, usually euthanasia must be taken into consideration [1].

The genomic profiling of canine PC is poorly explored. Few previous studies have evaluated the genomic of transcriptomic alterations in canine PC. In human, the molecular subtype of the PC is very important for the patient prognosis. The recurrent *SPOP*, FOXA1, and IDH1 mutations, genic fusions (*ERG*, *ETV1/4*, and FLI1), activated PI3K/AKT/mTOR and MAPK pathway mutations, and germ line or somatic DNA-repair gene mutations (including *BRCA1/2*, *CDK12*, *ATM*, *FANCD2*, and *RAD51C*) (~20% of primary PC) represent different subtypes of human PC [23].

Canine molecular alteration in E-cadherin, Caveolin-1, APC and β-catenin [24], NKX3.1 and c-Myc [3], c-KIT [25] and PTEN, TP53, MDM2, and AR expression [26] was previously described in literature. However, these studies have evaluated only gene expression. A recent study from our research group investigated the copy number alterations in canine PC [27]. We identified copy number loss in TP53 and PTEN and gain of MDM2, indicating the role of the TP53 pathway in the development of canine PC. Moreover, we identified many drug targets in canine PC, including VEGF and HER-2 (**Figure 7**) and imbalances in ILK signaling pathway (**Figure 8**).

Acknowledgements

The authors would like to thank Fundação de Amparo à Pesquisa do Estado de São Paulo (FAPESP) for its financial support (#2015/25400-7).

Conflict of interest

The authors have no conflict of interests.

Author details

Antonio Fernando Leis-Filho and Carlos E. Fonseca-Alves*
School of Veterinary Medicine and Animal Science, Sao Paulo State University—UNESP, Botucatu, Brazil

*Address all correspondence to: carloseduardofa@hotmail.com

References

[1] Smith J. Canine prostatic disease: A review of anatomy, pathology, diagnosis, and treatment. Theriogenology. 2008;**70**:375-383. DOI: 10.1016/j.theriogenology.2008.04.039

[2] Evans HE, Christensen GC. The urogenital system. In: Miller's Anatomy of the Dog. 4th ed. Philadelphia, USA: WB Saunders; 1993. pp. 514-516

[3] Fonseca-Alves CE, Kobayashi PE, Laufer-Amorim R. Evaluation of NKX3.1 and C-MYC expression in canine prostatic cancer. Research in Veterinary Science. 2018;**118**:365-370. DOI: 10.1016/j.rvsc.2018.04.001

[4] Fonseca-Alves CE, Gonçalves Corrêa A, Leal Santos-Junior H, Elias F, dos Santos Costa S, Dignani de Moura VMB. Abscesso prostático em cães: relato de 15 casos. Semina: Ciências Agrárias. 2012;**33**:1157-1164. DOI: 10.5433/1679-0359.2012v33n3p1157

[5] Lai CL, van den Ham R, van Leenders G, van der Lugt J, Teske E. Comparative characterization of the canine normal prostate in intact and castrated animals. The Prostate. 2008;**68**:498-507. DOI: 10.1002/pros.20721

[6] Dubé JY, Lazure C, Tremblay RR. Dog prostate arginine esterase is related to human prostate specific antigen. Clinical and Investigative Medicine. 1986;**9**:51-54

[7] Hayward SW, Cunha GR. The prostate: Development and physiology. Radiologic Clinics of North America. 2000;**38**:1-14. DOI: 10.1016/S0033-8389(05)70146-9

[8] Gobello C, Castex G, Corrada Y. Serum and seminal markers in the diagnosis of disorders of the genital tract of the dog: A mini-review. Theriogenology. 2002;**5**:1285-1291. DOI: 10.1016/S0093-691X(02)00628-3

[9] Barsanti JA, Finco DR. Canine prostatic diseases. Veterinary Clinics of North America: Small Animal Practice. 1986;**16**:587-599. DOI: 10.1016/S0195-5616(86)50063-2

[10] Korodi G, Igna V, Cernescu H, Mircu C, Frunză I, Knop R. Canine prostate pathology. Lucrari Stiintifice-Universitatea de Stiinte Agricole a Banatului Timisoara, Medicina Veterinara. 2008;**41**:187-194

[11] Sirinarumitr K, Johnston SD, Kustritz MVR, Johnston GR, Sarkar DK, Memon MA. Effects of finasteride on size of the prostate gland and semen quality in dogs with benign prostatic hypertrophy. Journal of the American Veterinary Medical Association. 2001;**218**:1275-1280. DOI: 10.2460/javma.2001.218.1275

[12] Paclikova K, Kohout P, Vlasin M. Diagnostic possibilities in the management of canine prostatic disorders. Veterinarni Medicina (Praha). 2006;**51**:1. DOI: 10.17221/5511-vetmed

[13] White RA. Prostatic surgery in the dog. Clinical Techniques in Small Animal Practice. 2000;**15**:46-51. DOI: 10.1053/svms.2000.7304

[14] Boland LE, Hardie RJ, Gregory SP, Lamb CR. Ultrasound-guided percutaneous drainage as the primary treatment for prostatic abscesses and cysts in dogs. Journal of the American Animal Hospital Association. 2003;**39**:151-159. DOI: 10.5326/0390151

[15] Lindberg R, Jonsson OJ, Kasström H. Sertoli cell tumours associated with feminization, prostatitis and squamous metaplasia of the renal tubular epithelium in a dog. Journal of Small Animal Practice. 1976;**17**:451-458. DOI: 10.1111/j.1748-5827.1976.tb06985.x

[16] Johnston SD, KamolpatanaK, Root-Kustritz MV, Johnston GR. Prostatic disorders in the dog.

Animal Reproduction Science. 2000;**60**:405-415. DOI: 10.1016/S0378-4320(00)00101-9

[17] De Marzo AM, Marchi VL, Epstein JI, Nelson WG. Proliferative inflammatory atrophy of the prostate: Implications for prostatic carcinogenesis. The American Journal of Pathology. 1999;**155**:1985-1992. DOI: 10.1016/S0002-9440(10)65517-4

[18] White RA, Williams JM. Intracapsular prostatic omentalization: A new technique for management of prostatic abscesses in dogs. Veterinary Surgery. 1995;**24**:390-395. DOI: 10.1111/j.1532-950X.1995.tb01349.x

[19] Bell FW, Klausner JS, Hayden DW, Feeney DA, Johnston SD. Clinical and pathologic features of prostatic adenocarcinoma in sexually intact and castrated dogs: 31 cases (1970-1987). Journal of the American Veterinary Medical Association. 1991;**199**:1623-1630

[20] Fonseca-Alves CE, Kobayashi PE, Rivera Calderón LG, Felisbino SL, Rinaldi JC, Drigo SA, et al. Immunohistochemical panel to characterize canine prostate carcinomas according to aberrant p63 expression. PLoS One. 2018;**12**:e0199173. DOI: 10.1371/journal.pone.0199173

[21] Gobello C, Corrada Y. Noninfectious prostatic diseases in dogs. Compendium on Continuing Education for the Practising Veterinarian-North American Edition. 2002;**24**:99-109

[22] Palmieri C, Grieco V. Proposal of Gleason-like grading system of canine prostate carcinoma in veterinary pathology practice. Research in Veterinary Science. 2015;**103**:11-15. DOI: 10.1016/j.rvsc.2015.09.004

[23] Cancer Genome Atlas Research Network. The molecular taxonomy of primary prostate cancer. Cell. 2015;**163**:1011-1025. DOI: 10.1016/j.cell.2015.10.025

[24] Kobayashi PE, Fonseca-Alves CE, Rivera-Calderón LG, Carvalho M, Kuasne H, Rogatto SR, et al. Deregulation of E-cadherin, β-catenin, APC and Caveolin-1 expression occurs in canine prostate cancer and metastatic processes. Research in Veterinary Science. 2018;**118**:254-261. DOI: 10.1016/j.rvsc.2018.03.004

[25] Fonseca-Alves CE, Kobayashi PE, Palmieri C, Laufer-Amorim R. Investigation of c-KIT and Ki67 expression in normal, preneoplastic and neoplastic canine prostate. BMC Veterinary Research. 2017;**13**:380. DOI: 10.1186/s12917-017-1304-0

[26] Rivera-Calderón LG, Fonseca-Alves CE, Kobayashi PE, Carvalho M, Drigo SA, de Oliveira Vasconcelos R, et al. Alterations in PTEN, MDM2, TP53 and AR protein and gene expression are associated with canine prostate carcinogenesis. Research in Veterinary Science. 2016;**106**:56-61. DOI: 10.1016/j.rvsc.2016.03.008

[27] Fonseca-Alves CE, Busso AF, Silveira SM, Rogatto SR, Amorim RL. Genomic gains in prostatic carcinoma and proliferative inflammatory atrophy in dogs. Cancer Research. 2014;**72**:5260. DOI: 10.1158/1538-7445.AM2012-5260

Chapter 6

Major Health Constraints and Ethno-Vet Practices of Small-Scale and Backyard Chicken Production in Some Selected Regions of Ethiopia

Meskerem Adamu Chere

Abstract

A study was conducted with the aim of assessing the major health constraints facing the small-scale and backyard chicken producers and ethno-vet practices exercised in five regions of the country: Amhara, Benishangul-Gumuz, Oromia, Southern region, and Tigray. Household respondents were purposively selected and interviewed. Data were collected through pretesting, semi-structural questionnaires, and field observation. The overall frequency of diseases reported as the main health constraint was Newcastle disease (64%) followed by gastrointestinal infection (34%), respiratory syndrome (22%), internal and external parasites (16%), coccidiosis (15%), and fowl pox (5%). They had no awareness how to manage chicken diseases (91.5%), and their flocks were not vaccinated (84%). High disease occurrence is reported in long rainy season (59%). Ethno-vet practice was experienced by the majority of the interviewed households (51.9%). A total of 19 medicinal plants were reported as being used as a traditional medicine. The main causes of losses were identified as disease (67%) and predator attack (32%). Poor disease prevention and control and the lack of knowledge and management skills were the major constraints of poultry production in the study areas. Research and extension efforts should be directed at the identified constraints. Farmer training and improvement of veterinary services are important.

Keywords: chicken, constraints, ethno-vet practices, small scale, backyard

1. Introduction

Poultry is the most widely used important species of animal in the majority of the countries, and it provides nutritionally beneficial food (animal protein); in addition, they can be raised with limited resources since they convert a scavenged feed resource into animal protein, and they are also used for generating income by the poor peri-urban and rural households [1]. According to the agricultural sample survey report of Central Statistical Authority [2] of 2014, the total chicken population in Ethiopia is estimated at about 51 million, of which 96.9, 2.4, and 0.8% are indigenous, hybrid, and exotic chickens, respectively. From these, 99%

IntechOpen

of them are reared under the traditional or scavenging production system of management, whereas 1% is reared under intensive management system [3, 4]. Above 98% of the total chicken products comes from village poultry [5, 6]. However, the production and productivity from village chickens are very low compared to their high numbers. This is mainly due to low productivity levels and poor management systems. There are also different constraints in the village chicken production systems. These include diseases, poor management, poor growth rates, predation, and lack of organized markets. Parasitic and other infectious diseases are also common in the tropics where the standard of husbandry is poor, and yet climatic conditions are favorable for the development of diseases [7, 8]. Poultry diseases are considered to be a serious problem for poultry production in Ethiopia. However management and health-care situations as well as ethno-vet practices are not adequately studied and compiled. The purpose of this study was, therefore, to develop a baseline information on management and major health constraints of chickens and ethno-vet practices in some selected parts of the country.

2. Research methodology

A survey study was conducted in five regional states of Ethiopia. Study regions have a relatively high density of chickens (**Figure 1**). Standing from the constraints of human labor and finance, purposive sampling method has been carried out to identify zones. Data were collected from a total of eight zones representing five regions, namely, Amhara (Debre Berhan and Kombolcha), Benishangul-Gumuz (Assosa), Oromia (Haramaya and Jimma), Southern region (Hawassa area and Yergalem), and Tigray (Mekelle), which are located in different agroecologies. Ethiopia has six traditional climatic zones, defined by altitude and temperature: (1) hot lowlands (<500 m), (2) lowlands (500–1500), (3) midlands (1500–2300), (4) highlands (2300–3200), (5) highlands (3200–3700), and (6) highlands (>3700). Except for Debre Berhan (2636) that is located at the highlands, most study areas are located at the midland climatic zones, Kombolcha (1825), Assosa (1514), Haramaya (2046), Jimma (1754), Hawassa area (1769), Yergalem (1735), and

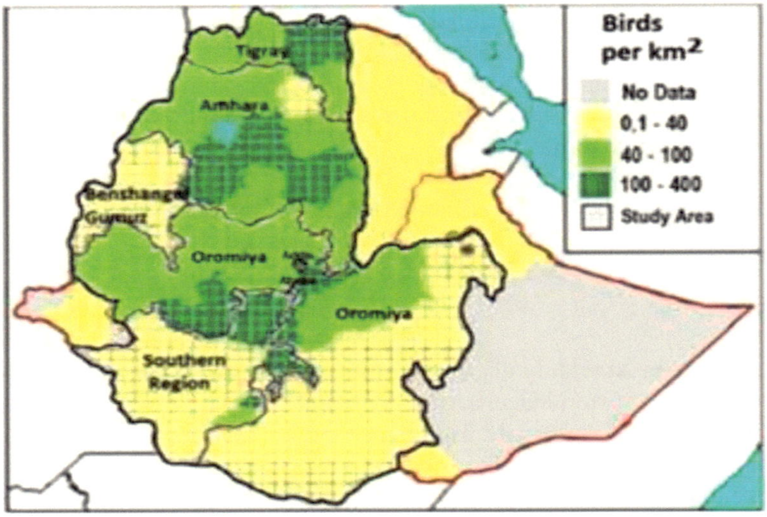

Figure 1.
Map of Ethiopia indicating poultry density and study area.

Questionnaire format used to assess major health constraints facing the small scale and backyard chicken producers and ethno-vet practices exercised in selected study areas of Ethiopia:

1: General Information:

1.1. Region________, Zone ________, District _______, Woreda/sub city ________ Name of enumerator _________ Signature_______

1.2. Name of Farmers or Managers___________

1.3. Education level: A. Illiterate B. Read and write C. Primary S, D. Secondary education, E. Higher education F. Training on chicken management G. Others

2. Chicken management: how many years have you risen chickens? _________

2.1. Housing systems: A. simple shade B. proper chicken house C. sharing with family

D. others _____________

2.2. What types of chicken breeds do you have? A. Exotic B. Hybrid (Crossbred) C. Local

2.3. Chicken flocks (Please indicate the number of chickens by their breed and age group)

S. N	Chicken age	Local	Crossbred	Exotic	Total
1	chicks (up to 8 weeks)				
2	growers (9 to 20 weeks)				
3	adult birds (more than 20 weeks)				

2.4. Who is responsible for chicken management?

A. Husband B. Wife C. Children E. Other (parent, neighbors, hired person), specify

3. Health:

3.1. Disease identification, mostly affected age, vaccination, treatment used, herbs or traditional medicines used, Awareness

S. N		Disease identification		Affected age	Vaccination		Treatment /vaccine type	Sources of drugs				Awareness	
1	number of sick chickens	local name/ symptom	scientific name		yes	no	Drugs /vaccine	herbs	Vet. clinic	human pharmacies	other	yes	no

3.2 Poultry disease: farmer's described diseases by symptoms and local names:

a) Noisy breathing, watery discharge from nose and coughing which spread rapidly in the flock. This was interpreted as respiratory syndrome or gunfan (local name).

b) Whitish green diarrhea, mass death, respiratory disease and paralysis, disease which could not be cured. This was interpreted as a Newcastle disease (fengil).

c) Acute respiratory disease of chickens characterized by nasal discharge, sneezing, and swelling of the face under the eyes. This was interpreted as Infectious choriza (yefit mabet).

d) Wart like lesions on the combs. And wattles that spread to the sides of the beaks. This was interpreted as fowl pox (fentata).

e) Passing out of bloody droppings, weakness, raffled feathers and lack of appetite. This was coccidiosis (yedem tekeimat).

f) Other

3.3. Do you treat? A. All your chickens B. Only sick chickens

3.4. Who administers the treatment? A. Farmers B. Animal health personnel

3.5. Do they cure after these treatments? A. Yes B. No C. sometimes yes

3.6. Have you ever lost all chickens due to diseases in the last 24 months? A. Yes B. No

If yes, what are the symptoms of diseases? ____________________

How many chickens due you lost? A. Quarter B. More than half

3.7. In which season do you observe high disease occurrence? Specify the disease type. Long rainy season = Jun, July, August and September. Short rainy season = February, March, April and May

A. Both in long & short rainy season B. Long rainy season C. Short rainy season.

3.8. What measure do you take during poultry disease outbreak?

A) Visit veterinary clinic ____ B) Sale infected bird's ___ C) Apply traditional medicine ___ D) Other options (mention)

3.9. What type of drugs/vaccine did you get from Veterinary clinic?

A. In form of powder B. Injectable drugs C. None D. vaccine

3.10. Have you ever bought any drug other than vet clinic? A. Yes B. no if yes, from where____

3.11. List down the names of traditional medicines you know or utilize for poultry disease treatment

A.________________ B.______________________ C.________________

3.12. Please indicate the part of plant materials used and mode of preparation________________

____

3.13. Have you ever lost all chickens due to predators in the last 24 months?

A. Yes B. No

3.14. How many chickens do you lost? A. Quarter B. More than half C. none

Figure 2.
A structured questionnaire used to select household respondents.

Mekelle (2143). The distance from the capital city, Addis Ababa and the study areas falls in the range 130 between and 783kms.

Two kebeles per zone with a high density of chickens and with known chicken-rearing practices were purposively selected in consultation with the respective agricultural development agencies. A total of 162 household respondents involved in small-scale and backyard chicken production (20 households in each zone) were selected and interviewed. Further information was also collected from individual observations and through open discussions during the time samples were collected.

There are local and exotic chicken breeds available in Ethiopia. Local (indigenous) chicken breeds are mostly called by their local name, which are named after the color of their feathers or their location. Exotic chickens are commercial breeds imported to Ethiopia for commercial purpose, either layers or broilers. Formerly the exotic ones were kept only in commercial farms with intensive management and the local or indigenous breeds in backyard or free-range chicken production systems. Currently, exotic and crossbreds (exotics with indigenous) are being kept in backyard chicken production systems with certain inputs [9]. According to FAO, the level of biosecurity in Ethiopian poultry production is classified into three: large commercial poultry production with "moderate to high biosecurity," small commercial poultry production with the "low to minimal" biosecurity, and village or backyard production with "minimal biosecurity" [10].

A structured questionnaire was carefully designed and administered to selected household respondents (**Figure 2**). The information inquired included general information, knowledge how to manage chickens, health care, health constraints, type and method of medicinal plants used to treat chicken disease, losses due to diseases, predator attack, etc. A single observation was made on chicken management and biosecurity, while a group discussion was used to identify diseases. Farmers describe diseases by their local name and symptoms that were previously defined in the questionnaire format.

The Statistical Analysis System (SAS) software [11] was used to enter and analyze the data. Descriptive statistics (mean, frequency and percentage) were also used to review the data.

3. Results

3.1 Chicken flock and house management

Of 162 household respondents, most of them kept local or indigenous chicken (49%) followed by indigenous and cross (42%) and exotic chicken breeds (8.8%). About 58% of the rural household respondents explained that they own chicken flocks between 4 and 15 birds, while the average was 9 birds/household. During this survey study, it was confirmed that about 33% of the household flock holdings ranged between 16 and 50 birds, while the average holding per a household was about 28 birds but exclusively hybrids. The holding size by the 8.8% was more than 50 birds, mainly exotic chicken with an average of 149 chicken flocks. Despite this, about 91% of households in the study area practiced free-range scavenging production system. The proportion of chicks and grower in the study flock samples was 24.5%, followed by adults about 18%, while adults and chicks together accounted for 57%.

Extra feed and water are rarely provided. This includes kitchen leftovers and some supplementary feeds. About 42% of chicken-rearing households explained that they

Factors	Category	Number of household respondents	Percent of household respondents
Breed	Local	78	49.05
	Local and cross	67	42.14
	Exotic	14	8.81
Flock size/average	4–15 (9)	92	57.8
	16–50 (28)	53	33.33
	51–300 (149)	14	8.81
Age group	Chicks and grower	39	24.53
	Adult	29	18.24
	Chicks and adult	91	57.23
House	Simple shade	66	41.51
	Shared with family	70	44.03
	Separate house	21	13.21
	Tree and roof	2	1.26
Care	Women	117	73.58
	Men	17	10.69
	Children	7	4.40
	Other	18	11.32

Table 1.
Flock and house management of small-scale and backyard chicken production.

keep their chickens in a simple shade, 44% of them share the same house with the chickens, 13% uses separate house, and 1% uses the birds to nest on the trees and roofs. According to a single visit done in some areas like Jimma, households kept chicks in haybox brooder during brooding time. About 74% of the respondents agreed that women are highly responsible for managing and caring the chickens, while 10.7% reported that men are responsible for the care of chickens. Children and other relatives also contribute in taking care of chickens for 4 and 11%, respectively (**Table 1**).

3.2 Disease occurrence

This study confirmed the prevalence of a number of poultry diseases. Farmers have thus reported a number of diseases based on clinical signs. Poultry diseases were previously described by their clinical sign and/or local names and then later translated to their scientific names (**Figure 3**). Newcastle disease is the most severe infectious disease reported. The overall frequency of Newcastle disease (NCD) occurrence was reported as 64%, gastrointestinal infection 34%, respiratory syndrome 22%, internal and external parasites 16%, coccidiosis 15%, and fowl pox 5%.

3.3 Village chicken health management

Of the interviewed village chicken households, 91.5% of the farmers had no awareness how to manage village chicken diseases. In the present study,

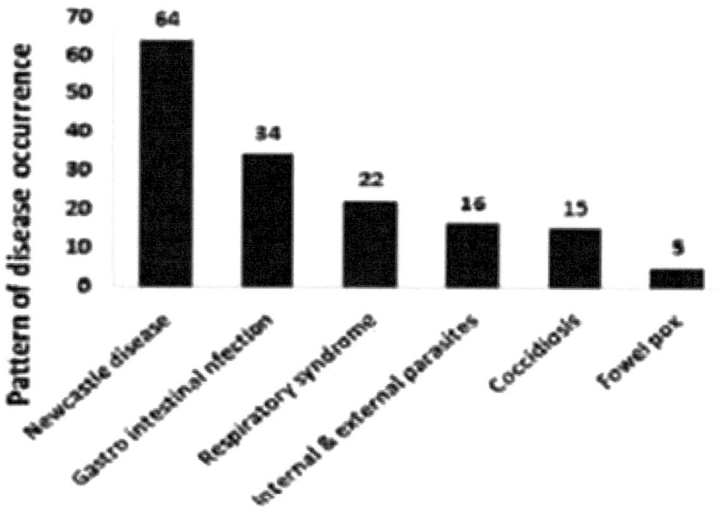

Figure 3.
Pattern of disease occurrence.

about 84% of household chicken flocks were not vaccinated. Some interviewed households (15.7%) reported that their chickens were vaccinated, but no routine vaccination campaigns against any poultry diseases are done by the official veterinary services to control backyard chicken diseases except to some outbreaks of Newcastle disease (**Table 2**).

Drugs and herbs used by village poultry household respondents during poultry disease outbreak to treat infected chickens were reported to be ineffective (55%) and sometimes effective (14.8%). Majority of village poultry households explained that they visit human pharmacy and/or apply traditional medicine (51%), while some of them visit veterinary clinic, sale infected birds, and do nothing during poultry disease outbreak.

3.4 Cause of chicken mortality and season of diseases occurrence

According to 29.6, 27, and 10% of the respondents, they replied that quarter, more than half, and all chickens died due to diseases, respectively, while 10, 13.8, and 8% of them replied that quarter, more than half, and all died due to predators attack, respectively (**Table 2**). Newcastle disease, respiratory diseases, and fowl pox outbreaks were reported to occur during the short rainy season: February, March, April, and May. Gastrointestinal infections, respiratory diseases, parasitic infestation, and coccidiosis were also frequently reported to occur during the long rainy season: June, July, August, and September. High disease occurrence was reported in long rainy season (59%).

3.5 The use of traditional poultry medicines

A total of 19 medicinal plants were reported as being used locally for the treatment of various chicken diseases as a traditional medicine. They use the leaf and the fruit (seeds) materials from the plant parts. The species of plants commonly used by smallholder farmers as a traditional medicine to treatscavenging chickens against some diseases are *Allium sativum*, *Allium cepa*, *Aloe vera*, *Azadirachta indica*, *Capsicum frutescens*, *Carica papaya*, *Citrus limon*, *Coffea arabica*, *Eucalyptus*

Parameters	Study areas								
	Amhara		Benishan-gulGumuz	Tigray	Southern region		Oromia		Over all
	Kombolcha	Debre Berhan	Asosa	Mekelle	Hawassa	Yirgalem	Jimma	Haramaya	
Awareness %									
Yes	27.7	7.1	0.0	10.5	10.0	4.8	0.0	7.7	8.5
No	72.2	92.9	100.0	89.5	90.0	95.2	100.0	92.3	91.5
Vaccination %									
No	50.0	100.0	90.0	63.2	90.0	80.9	100.0	100.0	84.3
Yes/none schedule	50.0	0.0	10	36.8	10.0	19.0	0.0	0.0	15.7
Treatment effect %									
Not effective	44.4	35.7	15.0	47.4	90.00	71.4	47.6	88.5	55.0
Effective	27.8	64.3	35.0	47.4	10.0	23.8	42.9	11.5	32.8
Sometimes effective	27.8	0.0	50.0	26.3	0.0	4.8	9.5	0.0	14.8
Proportion of sick chickens %									
No	5.6	7.1	5.0	26.3	35.0	28.6	14.3	34.6	19.5
Quarter	16.7	28.6	40.0	52.6	5.0	33.3	9.5	26.9	26.5
More than half	61.1	57.1	25.0	10.5	45.0	23.8	47.6	23.1	36.6
All	16.7	7.1	30.0	10.5	15.0	14.2	28.6	15.4	17.1
Mortality due to diseases %									
No	11.1	14.3	15.0	63.2	60.0	42.9	23.8	34.6	33.1
Quarter	16.7	35.7	55.5	21.0	15.0	38.0	23.8	30.8	29.6
More than half	55.6	42.9	20.0	5.3	15.0	9.5	42.9	26.9	27.3
All	16.7	7.1	10.0	10.5	10.0	9.5	9.5	7.7	10.1
Mortality due to predators %									
No	77.8	28.6	25.0	68.4	75.0	66.7	100.0	100.0	67.6
Quarter	16.7	14.3	25.5	15.8	5.0	4.8	0.0	0.0	10.2
More than half	5.6	35.7	30.0	10.5	15.0	14.2	0.0	0.0	13.8
All	0.0	21.4	20.0	5.3	5.0	14.2	0.0	0.0	8.2
Season of disease occurrence %									
Not known	16.7	0.0	0.0	10.5	0.0	0.0	0.0	0.0	3.4
Short/long rainy season	11.1	0.0	0.0	5.2	15.0	4.8	9.5	23.0	8.6
Short rainy season	33.3	7.1	80.0	10.5	25.0	28.6	23.8	23.1	28.9
Long rainy season	38.9	92.9	20.0	73.7	60.0	66.7	66.7	53.8	59.0

Table 2.
Chicken health management in selected areas of Ethiopia.

globulus, *Lantana camara*, *Lepidium sativum*, *Moringa stenopetala* and *Moringa oleifera*, *Nicotiana tabacum*, *Phytolacca dodecandra*, *Punica granatum*, *Ruta chalepensis*, *Vernonia amygdalina*, and *Zingiber officinale* (**Tables 3** and **4**). The main forms of administration are oral and local.

Family	Species	Disease/symptoms	Part used	Citation
Liliaceae	*Allium cepa* Linn	RD	Bulb	12
Liliaceae	*Allium sativum*	GID, NCD, and RD	Crushed bulb	40
Asphodelaceae	*Aloe vera* (L.)	Diarrhea, NCD, and RD	Leaf juice	5
Meliaceae	*Azadirachta indica*	Diarrhea	Leaf	25
Solanaceae	*Capsicum frutescens*	Diarrhea and NCD	Fruit	32
Caricaceae	*Carica papaya*	Coccidiosis and internal parasites	Leaf, fruit, and seed	10
Rutaceae	*Citrus limon* (L.)	Diarrhea and RD	juice	46
Rubiaceae	*Coffea arabica*	Diarrhea	Roasted and powdered coffee	7
Myrtaceae	*Eucalyptus globulus*	RD and depression	Fresh leaves	4
Verbenaceae	*Lantana camara*	White diarrhea	Fresh leaves	6
Brassicaceae Cruciferae	*Lepidium sativum*	Coccidiosis and diarrhea	Seed powder	40
Moringaceae	*Moringa oleifera*	Diarrhea and poor growth	Fresh leaves	6
Moringaceae	*Moringa stenopetala*	Diarrhea and poor growth	Fresh leaves	8
Solanaceae	*Nicotiana tabacum*	Skin problems (pox)	Fresh leaves	3
Phytolaccaceae	*Phytolacca dodecandra*	Skin problems (scabies)	Fresh leaves	6
Punicaceae	*Punica granatum*	Diarrhea, coccidiosis, and infectious diseases	Fresh leaves and fruits	5
Rutaceae	*Ruta chalepensis*	Diarrhea and depression	Fresh leaves	3
Asteraceae	*Vernonia amygdalina*	Diarrhea, coccidiosis, and GID	Fresh leaves	10
Zingiberaceae	*Zingiber officinale*	RD (cough/cold) and depression	Rhizome	10

GID, gastrointestinal disease; NCD, Newcastle disease; RD, respiratory disease.

Table 3.
Herbal medicines used to control village poultry diseases/symptoms in the study areas.

Zones	Species
Kombolcha	*Allium sativum*, *Allium cepa*, *Capsicum frutescens*, *Citrus limon*, *Lepidium sativum*, *Moringa*, *Punica granatum*
Debre Berhan	*Allium sativum*, *Allium cepa*, *Capsicum frutescens*, *Citrus limon*, *Lepidium sativum*, *Moringa*
Benishangul-Gumuz	*Allium sativum*, *Allium cepa*, *Carica papaya*, *Capsicum frutescens*, *Azadirachta indica*
Tigray	*Allium sativum*, *Allium cepa*, *Azadirachta indica*, *Capsicum frutescens*, *Citrus limon*, *Lepidium sativum*, *Moringa*, *Vernonia amygdalina*
Hawassa Zuria	*Allium sativum*, *Allium cepa*, *Azadirachta indica*, *Capsicum frutescens*, *Citrus limon*, *Eucalyptus globulus*, *Lepidium sativum*, *Moringa*, *Punica granatum*, *Ruta chalepensis*, *Vernonia amygdalina*
Yergalem	*Allium sativum*, *Capsicum frutescens*, *Citrus limon*, *Lepidium sativum*, *Ruta chalepensis*, *Zingiber officinale*
Jimma	*Allium sativum*, *Allium cepa*, *Capsicum frutescens*, *Citrus limon*, *Coffea Arabica*, *Lepidium sativum*, *Punica granatum*, *Vernonia amygdalina*, *Zingiber officinale*
Haramaya	*Allium sativum*, *Aloe vera*, *Capsicum frutescens*, *Citrus limon*, *Eucalyptus globulus*, *Lantana camara*, *Lepidium sativum*, *Phytolacca dodecandra*, *Punica granatum*, *Vernonia amygdalina*, *Zingiber officinale*

Table 4.
Herbal medicines reported in each zone.

4. Discussion

According to the present finding, most of the household respondents kept indigenous chicken (49%) followed by indigenous and cross (42%) and exotic chicken breeds (8.8%). These fall within the national agricultural sample survey report of Central Statistical Agency [2]. The report explains the distribution of the national chicken population comprising 96.9, 2.4, and 0.8% of indigenous, hybrid, and exotic chickens, respectively. About 58% of the rural household respondents explained that they own chicken flocks between 4 and 15 birds, while the average was 9 birds/household. This was consistent with the report of Tsegaw et al. [12] in the northwest part of Ethiopia, who reported flock size of 9 in the range of 2–30 birds per household. The holding size by 8.8% was more than 50 birds mainly exotic chicken with an average of 149 chicken flocks. This was observed in the urban and peri-urban areas, with households practicing small-scale semi-intensive and intensive production system. This is in agreement with the report of Demeke [10], who reported that intensive systems with a small number of exotic breeds of chicken (50–1000) are rising in the urban and peri-urban areas of the country, located in strategic areas close to market destinations. Despite this, about 91% of households in the study area practiced free-range scavenging production system. The proportion of chicks and grower in the study flock samples was 24.5%, followed by adults about 18%, while adults and chicks together accounted for 57%. Generally, most households kept chicken of all ages. These are in agreement with the observation of Sonaiya and Swan [13], who reported that free-range chicken flocks usually comprise different species of all ages.

It was found that management is generally poor, and extra feed and water are rarely provided. Village chickens scavenge most of the time. Households reported that they feed chickens with kitchen leftovers and some supplementary feeds including available cereal grains (maize, wheat, sorghum) and/or tubers. Housing of chickens varies widely depending on the chicken-rearing households.

This ranges from traditional housing made of grass and maize stalk to wire mesh fences. Chickens are enclosed and housed overnight in order to protect them from thieves and predators. On the other hand, during cropping season in the farming areas, the chickens are housed all day until harvesting in order to prevent them from destroying crops near the household and to protect them from predators. About 42% of chicken-rearing households explained that they keep their chickens in a simple shade, 44% of them share the same house with the chickens, 13% uses separate house and 1% uses the birds to nest on the trees and roofs. This was consistent with the previous result observed in north Gondar by Tsegaw et al. [12], who reported that 68% shares the main house or kitchen, 24% constructs separate shelter, while some birds (7%) perched in wooden materials or stayed overnight on a roof. According to a single visit done in some areas like Jimma, households kept chicks in haybox brooder during brooding time. However, management was generally poor; chicks were water soaked inside the hayboxes and thereby depressed. In order to minimize mortality of young chicks, the households in some areas of the study regions kept chicks close to the mother hens for some days. In terms of gender contribution, the women play the most significant role in feeding the chickens with kitchen leftovers and some supplementary feeds. About 74% of the respondents agreed that women are highly responsible for managing and caring the chickens.

The pattern of disease occurrence in free-range birds is different as opposed to incidences observed in intensive poultry production systems. Village chicken flocks usually consist of diverse species and all ages and are frequently close to the weather, environment, outbreaks of disease, and microorganisms and parasites found in the soil, wild birds, and animals [13]. Accordingly, this study confirmed the prevalence of a number of poultry diseases. Farmers have thus reported a number of diseases based on clinical signs. Newcastle disease is the most severe infectious disease reported. The overall frequency of Newcastle disease (NCD) occurrence was reported as 64%, gastrointestinal infection 34%, respiratory syndrome 22%, internal and external parasites 16%, coccidiosis 15%, and fowl pox 5%. These are supported by previous reports that are confirmed by several authors on backyard chicken flocks in Oromia region, Eastern Shewa (Gimbichu, Lume, and boset) woredas. Dagnachew [14] tested 328 blood samples and found Newcastle disease and fowl typhoid in 23.17 and in 22.87% of the samples, respectively. At the same time, also Yasmin [15] tested 327 blood samples and found mycoplasmosis in 64.5% of the samples. Mycoplasma species are known as the causative agent of chronic respiratory disease (CRD), synovitis, and airsacculitis. A possible explanation for the higher frequency of NCD in the areas of this study might be the difficulty of the local producers to identify NCD simply by the symptoms because NCD-causing virus species are so varied and cause various symptoms (nerves, respiratory, and digestive). Many other diseases also share the same symptoms which as result farmers may report other diseases as NCD. The disease is transmitted through droppings and secretions from the mouth, nose, and eyes of infected chicken. The disease can also spread through mechanical means like shoes, clothing, wild birds, etc. Mortality is more severe in young chickens than older chickens. However, egg production is severely reduced in older chickens [13].

In rural scavenging chicken flocks in those four districts of the Amhara Region, Eshetu et al. [16] also tested 267 fecal samples and found up to 9 different helminth parasites (nematode and cestoda) species in 91% of the samples. In Tiyo woreda, Arsi zone of the Oromia Region, Getachew et al. [17] tested 191 fecal samples from Rhode Island Red chicken breed and local chicken and found coccidian oocysts in 80.7 and 61% of samples, respectively, while Adamu [18] tested fecal samples from a respective of 88 and 12 small- and large-scale broiler farms located in Central Ethiopia (Debre Zeit, Dukem, Mojo, and Nazareth towns) and found coccidian oocysts in 60% of the farms.

Of the interviewed village chicken households, 91.5% of the farmers had no awareness how to manage village chicken diseases. In general, similar problems were observed on village chicken health management system across all regions. In the present study, about 84% of household chicken flocks were not vaccinated against any poultry diseases. This might be due to the lack of awareness and the difficulty on accessing and handling the vaccine in free-range family chicken production systems. The vaccine dosage may not match to the village chicken flock sizes, which is mostly less than 50 birds; in addition, the lack of basic infrastructure and maintenance of the cold chain in some remote areas is difficult. Some interviewed households (15.7%) reported that their chickens were vaccinated against some outbreaks of Newcastle disease. However, no routine vaccination campaigns are done by the official veterinary services to control backyard chicken diseases. In general, vaccination management and disease control method in the free-range family chicken production systems are difficult (**Table 2**).

Compared to small-scale semi-intensive and intensively kept commercial chickens, drugs and herbs used by village poultry household respondents during poultry disease outbreak to treat infected chickens were reported to be ineffective (55%) and sometimes effective (14.8%). They complain about the ineffectiveness of some of those drugs or herbs used for the treatment of infected chickens or for the control of mortality. This might be due to the absence of vaccination practices (unless vaccinated, viral diseases are incurable), the application of none standardized drugs (drugs prepared for human, unknown dose application, and the use of combination of many drugs or herbal medicines). The veterinary drugs and veterinary service insufficiencies in remote areas and the high cost of veterinary drugs were also reported. Majority of village poultry households explained that they visit human pharmacy and/or apply traditional medicine (51%), while some of them visit veterinary clinic, sale infected birds, and do nothing during poultry disease outbreak.

According to 29.6, 27, and 10% of the respondents, they replied that quarter, more than half, and all chickens died due to diseases, respectively, while 10, 13.8, and 8% of them replied that quarter, more than half, and all died due to predators attack, respectively, in the last 24 months (**Table 2**). However, differences on the rates of mortality were recorded among regions; this agreed with findings of Gueye [19], who reported that farm poultry production systems are related to high mortality (mainly due to Newcastle disease), in tropical Africa. Disease patterns vary according to the season. Newcastle disease is more serious during the dry season [13]. In the present study, household respondents also reported the occurrence of Newcastle disease, respiratory diseases, and fowl pox outbreaks during the short rainy season and the occurrence of gastrointestinal infections, respiratory diseases, parasitic infestation, and coccidiosis in the long rainy season.

Traditional medicine like herbal therapies are widely used by the majority of African people to treat various human and animal diseases, and it is the only choice for most of them since veterinarians working in African rural areas almost remain inaccessible [20]. Most village farmers in the study regions depend on herbal remedies for indigenous poultry health management. A total of 19 medicinal plants were reported as being used locally for the treatment of various chicken diseases as a traditional medicine. They use the leaf and the fruit (seeds) materials from the plant parts. The application is in the form of juice from freshly collected leaves or in the form of powder from dried seeds. The remedies are prepared by grinding both the leaves and the seeds. These herbal medicines can be prepared in a single or combination of two or three herbs. Of 19 reported medicinal plants, *Allium sativum*, *Capsicum frutescens*, *Citrus limon*, *Lepidium sativum*, and *Azadirachta indica* were the most frequently used herbs. However, the dosage applications are not consistent.

5. Conclusion

The main causes of losses were identified as disease and predator attack. Poor disease prevention and control and the lack of knowledge, management skills, and provision of feed, water, and housing were also identified as the major constraints of poultry production in the study areas. Newcastle disease is the most severe infectious disease reported by the farmers followed by gastrointestinal infection, respiratory syndrome, internal and external parasites, coccidiosis, and fowl pox. During poultry disease outbreak, households reported that they visit human pharmacy and/or apply herbal medicines; however, there is no scientific document available which proves the efficacy and the dosage administration of the medicinal plants or human medicines used to control poultry diseases. Farmers reported the ineffectiveness of some drugs or herbs. No routine vaccination campaigns against any poultry diseases are done by the official veterinary services to control backyard chicken diseases except to some outbreaks of Newcastle disease. Some of small-scale commercial poultry farms located in and around urban and semi-urban areas practiced vaccination program. The free-range management systems make vaccination of chickens difficult. The pattern of disease occurrence varies according to the season. In the present study, household respondents reported the occurrence of Newcastle disease, respiratory diseases, and fowl pox outbreaks during the short rainy season. On the other hand, gastrointestinal infections, respiratory diseases, parasitic infestation, and coccidiosis were reported to occur in the long rainy season. A total of 19 medicinal plants were reported as being used locally for the treatment of various chicken diseases. Better feeding, watering, hygiene, and protection management and control of diseases and mortality are important methods to improve indigenous chicken production at household level. Family chicken producers should be trained on how to improve housing, nutrition, and disease control practices. They should also be supported and experienced on how to reduce the identified constraints through improved biosecurity and vaccination against diseases such as NCD. Efforts should be made to make the delivery of heat-stable and easily administered vaccines and drugs to these remote areas easier and to verify the effectiveness and the dosages of some traditionally used herbal medicines. The veterinary services need to be strengthened to control indigenous chicken diseases at household level. Research and extension efforts should be directed at the identified constraints.

Acknowledgements

This study is part of a project entitled “Improving Productivity and Value Addition in Non-Ruminant Livestock: Development and Promotion of Poultry Production Technologies,” which is funded by the Debre Zeit Agricultural Research Center (DZARC) under the Ethiopian Institute of Agricultural Research (EIAR). The author is grateful to all.

Conflict of interest

There is no conflict of interest to declare.

Author details

Meskerem Adamu Chere
Ethiopian Biotechnology Institute, Addis Ababa, Ethiopia

*Address all correspondence to: mesku12345@yahoo.com

References

[1] Van Eekeren N, Maas AS, Verschuur HWM. Small-Scale Chicken Production. Wageningen: Agromisa Foundation and CTA; 2006. pp. 6-91

[2] Central Statistical Agency (CSA). Statistical Bulletin 573: Agricultural Sample Survey Report on Livestock and Livestock Characteristics. Vol. II. Addis Ababa, Ethiopia; 2014

[3] Ashenafi H, Eshetu Y. Study on gastrointestinal helminthes of local chickens in Central Ethiopia. Revue de Médecine Vétérinaire. 2004;**155**:504-507

[4] Tadelle D, Kijora C, Peters KJ. Indigenous chicken ecotypes in Ethiopia: Growth and feed utilization potentials. International Journal of Poultry Science. 2003;**2**:144-152

[5] Tadelle D. Studies on village poultry production systems in the central highlands of Ethiopia [thesis]. Uppsala, Sweden: Swedish University of Agriculture Sciences; 1996

[6] Udo HMJ, Asgedom AH, Viets TC. Modeling the impact of interventions in village poultry systems. Agricultural Systems. 2006;**88**:255-269

[7] Hailemariam T, Legesse D, Alemu Y, Negusse D. Adopting poultry breeds in the highlands of Ethiopia. In: Research Report. Ethiopian Institution of Agricultural Research; 2006. p. 65

[8] Tadesse G. Investigations into technical interventions to improve rural poultry production systems in South Wello Zone [thesis]. Ethiopia: Alemaya University; 2005

[9] USAID UGP, Urban Gardens Program 2012. Assessment of available chicken breeds in Ethiopia; July 2012

[10] Demeke S. Animal Production and Health Division, Emergency Centre for Transboundary Animal Diseases, Socio Economics, Production and Biodiversity Unit: Poultry Sector Country Review: An Analysis of the Poultry Sector in Ethiopia. Rome, Italy: FAO; 2008

[11] SAS: Statistical Analysis System. The 2003 SAS Online Doc. 9.1.3. Cary, NC, USA: SAS Institute Inc

[12] Tsegaw F, Birhanu A, Tesfu K. Small-scale family poultry production in North Gondar: Characteristics, productivity and constraints. In: Livestock Research for Rural Development. 2013. p. 25

[13] Sonaiya EB, Swan SEJ. Small-scale poultry production. Animal Production and Health Manual. Rome: FAO; 2004

[14] Dagnachew B. Characterization of village chicken production system with emphasis on selected health problems in eastern Shoa zone, Oromia [thesis]. Faculty of Veterinary Medicine Debre Zeit, Addis Ababa University; 2007

[15] Yasmin J. Cross sectional study and isolation of Mycoplasma gallisepticum in commercial and backyard chickens in East Showa, Ethiopia [thesis]. Faculty of Veterinary Medicine Debre Zeit Ethiopia, Addis Ababa University; 2007

[16] Eshetu Y, Mulualem E, Ibrahim H, Berhanu A, Aberra K. Study of gastro-intestinal helminths of scavenging chickens in four rural districts of Amhara region, Ethiopia. Revue Scientifique et Technique (International Office of Epizootics). 2001;**20**:791-796

[17] Getachew G, Getachew T, Dorchies PH. Study on poultry coccidiosis in Tiyo District, Arsi zone, Ethiopia. International Journal of Poultry Science. 2008;7:251-256

[18] Adamu M. Evaluation of risk factors associated with coccidiosis in broiler farms of selected towns of Ethiopia. African Journal of Basic & Applied Sciences. 2015;**7**:34-40

[19] Gueye EF. Family poultry research and development in low-income food-deficit countries: Approaches and prospects. Outlook on Agriculture. 2002;**31**:13-21

[20] Gueye EF. Ethnoveterinary medicine against poultry diseases in African villages. World's Poultry Science Journal. 1999;**55**

Section 4

Exotics Wildlife and Conservation

Chapter 7

Veterinarian's Role in Conservation Medicine and Animal Welfare

Diana Raquel Neves Fernandes
and Maria de Lurdes Ribeiro Pinto

Abstract

The enhanced role of human actions brings new escalating conservation challenges and emerging diseases, which pressure impaired long-term survival of threatened free-ranging and captive wildlife species, while having hazardous effects on ecosystems and public health. Veterinarians have not only a broad education in comparative medicine (not a single-species focus) but also are also highly trained in recognizing, diagnosing and understanding disease impact on public health as well as on individuals, populations and whole ecosystems. Their skills and expertise turns them into valuable key players in planning, implementing and effectively assisting both in-situ and ex-situ conservation projects. In parks and zoological gardens, major goals have now won priority: the conservation of worldwide fauna and flora and the protection of animal welfare. Today, animal welfare can be scientifically assessed to determine the quality of life of individuals, in which behavioral assessment and behavioral enrichment are fundamental tools.

Keywords: veterinary, conservation medicine, zoological institutions, animal welfare, animal behavior, behavioral enrichment

1. Introduction

Current extinction rates are outstandingly high (about 1000 times previously valued ones) and likely to be underestimated once biodiversity statistics are affected by a gap of information on species taxonomy, distribution and status [1]. The enhanced role of human actions brings new escalating conservation challenges and emerging diseases, which pressure impaired long-term survival of threatened free-ranging and captive wildlife species, while having hazardous effects on ecosystems and public health [2–4]. Biodiversity conservation currently requires a broader approach, capable of connecting interdisciplinary bridges between the diversity of social, economic, political and biological variables which influence health issues, so to understand their complex interaction and therefore find new solutions bearing in mind human and animal well-being while preserving ecosystems, in what is designated as the "OneHealth" approach. Zoological and wildlife medicine are acknowledged scientific branches within the veterinary profession, which emerged in the 1990s as a response to increasing concerns regarding wildlife protection, and that now fully integrate the transdisciplinary frame that characterizes Conservation Biology [2]. Wildlife veterinarians and the zoological community have a pivotal role to play in the future of biodiversity conservation as, apart from saving numbers of species and understanding the consequences of animal diseases to human communities, they also encompass the protection of functional and integrated ecosystems, applying their skills and scientific knowledge on the emerging field of Conservation Medicine [5, 6].

Modern zoos and aquariums have a responsibility towards the animals under their protection, through their whole life stages. Captivity can affect drastically animal behavior. By confining animals to a cage or enclosure, we reduce the complexity of their environment, severely narrowing the natural control they should detain over it and restricting the range of behaviors they are able to exhibit [7]. Where animals have very limited choices we are the ones planning almost all aspects of their life (e.g., feeding schedules, what to eat, where to sleep, who to live or to reproduce with). Effects of sensory deprivation and physical variety in the environment may result in aggression, boredom, anxiety, frustration and, ultimately, both physical and physiological illness [8]. Furthermore, preservation of core biological behaviors is essential [to the survival of the individuals targeted for release and reintroduction in the wild and, therefore, for the success of conservation programs [9] Thus, captive establishments have an ethical and legal obligation to provide for the holistic welfare of all animals under their protection. They should work in an organized way in order to achieve high standards of animal welfare (AW), comply with animals' wide range of needs and minimize the incidence of negative states while promoting positive ones [10]. This involves providing: (1) appropriate, safe and naturalistic environments; (2) proper diet; (3) adequate veterinary care; (4) appropriate social contact and (5) environmental enrichment [10, 11]. Overall assessment AW is by no means straightforward and should be carried out in a scientific and objective way, avoiding anthropomorphism and taking no account of ethical topics about the practices or conditions being compared in its evaluation [12, 13].

2. Wildlife veterinarians and conservation medicine

In the past, the primary role of wildlife veterinarians was the intervention and management of free-ranging populations experiencing a health crisis [14]. Epidemic wildlife disease was mainly addressed due to its zoonotic menace (e.g., rabies, brucellosis and tuberculosis) and its harmful outcome in the health of domestic animals or game species considered economically relevant [14, 15]. In the meantime, veterinarians from zoological institutions focused on the *ex-situ* individual, providing healthcare and ensuring compliance of welfare criteria for captive collections while their main part in wildlife conservation projects was considered to be the chemical immobilization of animals in order to enable research [4, 15]. Presently, differences in the role of wildlife and zoo veterinarians are fading as a result of the expansion of the role of the latest in conservation efforts. Such tendency was inevitable due to marked changes in zoo's missionary priorities and an increase in the movement of animals between facilities or for intended release in the wild [2, 3]. When it comes to decide whether to prioritize the interests or rights of animals individually or to focus on the global viability and health of populations and species in specific situations zoological veterinarians are those in the best position to offer a balanced view concerning what the best is for the animals, either from an individual or population perspective. They are expected to actively promote and safeguard animal welfare on the grounds of scientifically justified practices which encompasses a wide range of medical activities, summarized in **Table 1** [16].

2.1 Zoological institutions' evolution and current missions

Zoological institutions have served many different purposes and undergone a remarkable evolution throughout the years until the present days. The first

- Health assessment, surveillance and log-term monitoring for feral and domestic animal populations within park borders
- Identification of critical health factors with impact on wildlife population dynamics
- Development and enforcement of new health care technologies and methodologies
- Provision of preventive, diagnostic and therapeutic health care for wildlife species
- Improvement of safety and efficiency of methods of animal handling and secure addressing of other ethical and welfare concerns
- Active participation and inspection of zoological management decisions such as husbandry, nutrition, animal shipment and pest control
- Scientific biological data collection, analysis and management
- Active participation in captive breeding programs
- In situ and ex-situ reproductive and health management of threatened species
- Disease risk analysis and creation of health screening and quarantine protocols for wildlife translocation projects
- Management of emerging disease and health crisis intervention
- Research on zoonotic, anthropozoonotic and interspecies transmission of disease
- Interdisciplinary collaboration in conservative efforts
- Guidelines and policy development at local, national and international levels
- Training of field personnel to expand their skills in addressing wildlife health issues

Table 1.
Applied veterinary medicine and research in supporting both ex-situ and in-situ conservation programs.

models of modern zoos emerged during 18th century, a period known as "Age of Enlightenment" and characterized by educational and scientific endeavors such as animal behavior and anatomy research, which brought a new perspective and goal to the outdated "Menageries" [17]. In the 1970s public opinion began to change and society become more sensitive to the ethical concepts of environmental and animal welfare, leading to the emergence of movements which drove zoos to develop new intentional statements. Such intentions would emphasize the conservation of endangered species, animal welfare and more naturalistic exhibits' construction, turning the entertainment of visitors into a secondary objective [18].

In this day and age, modern zoos have a far more important role and are beyond the old tight and empty iron barred cages with concrete floors. Despite the fact that they are still profitable and recreational centers, they are now driven by a new set of missions and ethical principles: education and public awareness, scientific research, and reproduction/conservation of endangered species along with the preservation of their habitats [19, 20]. In order to overcome a still widespread infamous reputation which infers that zoos are prisons, holding captive animals for the amusement of humans in conditions which are fully inadequate to ensure their quality of life [21], it is imperative that these missions establish an ethical commitment to one another, so they can ensure the well- being of the animals intended to protect.

Currently, there are a number of institutions which follow a professional code of ethics and are responsible for accrediting modern zoos as well as promoting program coordination and cooperation between zoological gardens and aquariums worldwide. They provide its members with services that meet the highest standards and best practices in animal care, and support scientific research, conservation, and public engagement [22]. The World Association of Zoos and Aquariums (WAZA), for example, is the unifying organization of the zoological community (including more than 300 members) and the founding member of IUCN [23]. All member institutions have established Taxon Advisory Groups (TAG) for all the different species of animals that are kept in zoos and aquariums. Each TAG focuses on the sustainability and conservation needs of an entire taxa and develops a Regional Collection Plan accordingly, which identifies essential conservative and research goals, develops an action plan and liberates specific recommendations for ex situ and in situ population management [23]. TAG's are composed by professional specialists who are also responsible for advising, managing and supporting cooperative animal management programs like Species Survival Plans (SSP), European Endangered species Programs (EEP) and international Studbooks (SB) [11, 22]. Most endangered species are part of cooperative international and scientifically managed breeding programs whose final goal is to sustain populations that are healthy, genetically viable, demographically stable and capable of self-reproduction, so they can serve as a "gene pool" and surplus for eventual reintroduction in their natural habitat [24, 25].

Accredited zoological institutions ought to have veterinary clinicians working closely with a variety of other institution's organizational staff (such as animal care providers; endocrinology, behavioral or nutritional field specialists; ecologists; regulatory board of directors; and even educational, marketing or facility design departments) and who actively participate in management decisions [2, 15]. Clear communication among the different interest groups existing within a zoological institution allows for the creation of holistic medical programs whose lead foundation is preventive medicine and through which animals can be regarded as one population/community, while still having their individual needs attended [26]. Keeper staff should be trained for clinical health assessment, so they could be better qualified at understanding, identifying and promptly reporting any signs of injury or abnormal behavior that could indicate early disease stages [2]. All data collected and medical records should be condensed in databases like Medical Animal Record Keeping System (MedARKS) or Zoological Information Management System (ZIMS), for cooperative consultancy of disease occurrence and share of information between institutions at a global level. A standardized, computerized medical record-keeping system is a useful tool for management of health care and husbandry practices. By documenting and analyzing medical information that is easily assessed (e.g., clinical notes, treatments, anesthesia, parasitology) it can help future disease assessment or comparison with other populations [27]. Complete reports of necropsies on collection animals should be kept as well, once they can provide information about species anatomy that has great value for surgical procedures.

One of the most exalted contributions of the zoological veterinarian nowadays is its aid in successful captive breeding programs. Apart from securing animal general health, the veterinarian is able to access reproductive health and behavior, monitor breeding cycles, establish management protocols, help in implementing artificial reproductive techniques and effectively control selective reproduction, with resource to permanent or reversible contraceptive methods [2, 3, 14, 15]. Despite the practical and financial difficulties inherent to breeding programs [28], the extremely small capacity of zoos and the relatively uncommon and unsuccessful levels of reintroduction of propagated species, one must not depreciate the importance of zoo's conservative efforts and its ability to reproduce key species which have no other preservation options [5]. In recent years, zoos have bred about 19% of all known mammals' species and at least 9% of the birds [28]. International Studbooks are documents where all records and data relevant to the whole captive population of a certain species integrated in a breeding program, are compiled and continuously updated [23]. They will provide vital information on pedigree and breeding history of individual animals along with several changes in captive populations, and they will assist with references on pairing choices in order to ensure the maximal genetic diversity within the population. These references will recommend which individuals should breed with whom, how often and where [23, 29, 30]. Studbooks also recommend breeding restrictions in order to avoid future uncontrolled population expansion and therefore achieve stability [24, 30].

3. Veterinarians' role in animal welfare and behavioral assessment

The veterinary works under an ethical code of professional conduct which implies a commitment with integrated principles of animal welfare and the individual responsibility of ensuring a rational enforcement of the "Five Freedoms" (**Table 2**). All animals must be treated with respect, dignity and compassion as well as with thoughtful consideration for their species-typical biology and behavior [31]. Despite significant advances concerning the animal welfare (AW) topic through recent years, the majority of the research conducted has involved farm and domesticated animals [32, 33]. Zoological collections still include many poorly understood species as well as individuals with different life experiences and particular temperaments [32]. Animal welfare is a wide multi-disciplinary concept for which many definitions have been proposed. Animal welfare as a scientific field started with the Brambell Report on the welfare of intensively farmed animals, issued by the British government in 1965 [34] and later revised by the Farm Animal Welfare Council (FAWC) in 1979, having resulted in the decree of five formalized and rightful freedoms that would form a logical and comprehensive framework for analysis of animal welfare [35]. Farm Animal Welfare Council claims that the welfare of an animal includes both its physical fitness and mental state and that "any animal kept by man, must at least, be protected from unnecessary suffering". Webster [36] considers that although the "absolute attainment of all five freedoms is unrealistic", they still represent an "attempt to make the best of a complex and difficult situation". Some of these freedoms, like the freedom from fear and distress or freedom from pain, are anthropocentric constructs. Fear and pain are normal and essential in appropriate situations, where they work as natural defense mechanisms and may have adaptive and fitness value [37]. Conclusively, the freedoms define "ideal states rather than standards for acceptable welfare" [35] and are best viewed as useful and practical principles that provide the basic philosophy to minimize suffering and promote a state of good welfare and assessment of any husbandry system.

Today, AW can be scientifically assessed to determine the quality of life of individuals, and it implies the integration of the animal's biological function, as well as the subjective emotions and sensations it experiences as a result of the surrounding environment [10]. Consequently, the individual's health is highlighted as a "state of complete physical, mental and social well-being and not merely the absence of disease or infirmity" [38]. Broom [39] also utters that "The welfare of an individual is

1. **Freedom from hunger and thirst**—by ready access to fresh water and a diet to maintain full health and vigor
2. **Freedom from discomfort**—by providing an appropriate environment including shelter and a comfortable resting area
3. **Freedom from pain, injury or disease**—by prevention or rapid diagnosis and treatment
4. **Freedom to express normal behavior**—by providing sufficient space, proper facilities and company of the animal's own kind
5. **Freedom from fear and distress**—by ensuring conditions and treatment which avoid mental suffering

Table 2.
The "Five Freedoms" which constitute the primary basic principles for animal welfare.

its state as regards its attempts to cope with its environment". Welfare is, therefore, a characteristic of an individual [8, 12] and will vary on a dimensional continuum from very poor to very good [10, 37] as a measure of the animal's perception of its external circumstances and lived experiences [40]. The ability of an organism to tolerate and respond to a range of stimulation, including noxious stimuli, in order to maintain mental and body stability, is called "Coping" [32]. Coping implies the concepts of homeostasis and adaptation, as well as brain activity, endocrine, immunological, physiological and behavioral complex response mechanisms [8]. Scientific consideration of subjective emotional states in AW has been disregarded since these are difficult to identify and quantify [32, 37]. However, active promotion of positive feelings, such as pleasure and contentment, plays a primary role in assuring good welfare status [8, 41] provided that this is determined from an overall balance of experiences. Addressing only the negative emotions and states will not necessarily give rise to positive ones but will merely serve to achieve a neutral situation [10, 40]. Animals have a wide range of needs, which must be always met appropriately according to each species and based on scientific principles, so as to minimize negative welfare states while promoting positive ones [10]. Failure or difficulty to cope with the environment occurs together with the presence of negative emotional states (suffering) and subjective experiences, and it represents a state of poor welfare, from a holistic view of well-being [12, 42]. Animals seek to control interactions with their environment and avoid unpleasant stimuli. When unable to do so, and simultaneously denied resources they are very strongly motivated to obtain, they will achieve a distressful state of frustration and anxiety [10, 43]. Stress is currently defined by its consequences and described as detrimental as a reaction to a challenging stimuli that will activate the organism's hypothalamus-pituitary-adrenal (HPA) axis and produce a response with adverse effects that disrupts homeostasis [8], resulting in overall reduced fitness [32]. It can lead to a variety of short and long term responses characterized by a range of physiological abnormalities (i.e., alterations in hormonal profiles, metabolic changes and cardiovascular malfunction) [8] as well as psychological disorders (maladaptive demeanor such as increased occurrence of pacing, aggression, self-mutilation or fear behaviors) [43]. It is therefore essential to provide animals with productive environments that reward them with fresh challenges, opportunities and choices over time which allow them to express innate behavior and control interactions with their surroundings [8, 10]. Animals are now acknowledged as "sentient beings" [44], considered to have value of their own and to be able of conscious feeling and subjectively perceiving both positive and negative emotions and experiences. Despite the whole concept of AW involving moral values and judgments about our obligations to the animals under our care, it is only after scientific evidence on welfare assessment has been obtained that ethical questions and decisions are ought to be taken [8, 12]. Qualitative and quantitative scientific methods for determining acceptable high standards of AW are complex and multidisciplinary [32] and involve indirect (by taking into consideration the animal needs) and direct measurement of variables, both conducted through observation and experimentation. It is imperative that a variety of "welfare indicators" are used [12] in order to obtain a comprehensive view of the animal's biological state which is characterized by several interacting components that result in neural, endocrine, sensory, immunological and behavioral responses when faced with challenge [8]. WAZA recommends that zoos and aquariums apply a simple "Five Domains" model to facilitate the assessment and understanding of AW, which schematically outlines four functional domains (i.e., "nutrition", "environment", "physical health" and "behavior") and one "Mental" domain. This useful model links a variety of internal/external conditions with the negative (aversive) or positive (pleasant) experiences they give rise to, and integrates its effects in order to draw the sketch of a welfare status [10]. Some physiological indices cannot be obtained safely in non-trained zoo animals without the use of anesthesia or sedatives (e.g., changes in heart and respiratory rates, blood parameters, hormonal profiles or neurotransmitters' levels) [8]. Alternatively, other internal parameters can be collected noninvasively, for example, measuring reproductive or stress hormones and their metabolites in urine or feces (e.g., fecal estrogens or fecal glucocorticoids) [12, 32]. The HPA axis' frequent and high activity is the most often used physiologic measure [32], very useful in assessing stress responses and impaired immune system associated with environmental disturbance. It is usually monitored noninvasively through analysis of fecal cortisol/corticosterone [42, 45]. Although efforts should be made to include the importance of both positive (pleasure, contempt) and negative feelings or sensations (suffering, fear, pain) in the assessment of AW, these imply complex brain constructs and functioning mechanisms which are not easy to evaluate in a fully objective way [8]. Dawkins [43] argues that animal welfare should be assessed by answering two essential questions: (1) Are the animals healthy? and (2) Do they have what they want?, and that these two queries concentrate both the physical and the mental features of AW. Some indirect methods that help answering these key questions and are frequently used for AW assessment and improvement, include behavioral observation associated with tests that identify individuals' choices/preferences or study their motivational strength by "asking" the animals what they want and how much they want it. The way an animal responds to given opportunities in its environment offers valuable information about its emotional state and motivation, and helps to determine a particular hierarchy of needs [40, 45].

Animal welfare is considered to be a scientific branch of applied animal behavior and may be measured through behavioral assessment [46]. Understanding behavioral diversity, its function and its relation with the animal's perception of their external circumstances is important as it might help to prevent what is considered an abnormal demeanor or to improve conditions that are appropriate for normal repertoires. Skinner [47] considers that behavior is "part of the total activity of an organism" and that "is that part of the functioning organism which is engaged in acting upon or having commerce with the outside world". Behavior as a specific response, therefore represents the first line of defense to environmental challenging stimuli and may delineate a rough sketch of an animal's coping success against external stressors [10, 42]. It plays a major role in answering Dawkin's [43] questions: (1) "Are the animals healthy?" and (2) "Do they have what they want?", since it encompasses animals' own decision-making process and represents a phenotypic expression of emotions [43] while it also may be used in the clinical assessment of animal's health status (e.g., assessment of pain, nutritional requirements and hormonal conditions) [43, 48]. Behavior assessment through applied behavior analysis and behavioral monitoring studies is a technique that has several benefits supporting optimal animal care, making it essential to improve animal welfare and to meet conservation goals. These studies have emphasis on scientific data collection through direct and objective observation of measurable behavior as well as the circumstances under which they occur, and concern the functional relationships between environment and expressions of behavior [43, 48]. Systematic observations and record keeping have numerous advantages as a management tool in zoos and other related facilities: they represent a non-invasive and, in the majority of cases, a non-intrusive technique [43] that allows documentation of normal behavior patterns and identification of any changes on regular activity, establishing a database of background information on individuals on a consistent basis [48].

3.1 Behavioral enrichment

The History of enrichment starts in the 1920s with Robert Mearns Yerkes [49], a psychobiologist best known for his work in intelligence testing of both humans and primates and his writings about the importance of enrichment for gorillas and chimpanzees in captivity [50]. The Swiss zoologist Heini Hediger (1908–1992), known as the "father of zoo biology", was a visionary in the proxemics in animal behavior. In the 1950s, and for the next several decades, he wrote about human responsibility in providing constructive environments for wild animals in zoos and described the importance of studying animal's territorial surroundings, having a particular influence on the construction and planning of naturalistic enclosures [49, 51]. His revolutionary concepts are well expressed in his book in which he refers that "Anyone who sets out to build homes for animals should be quite clear that the cube is the most unbiological and therefore most inappropriate of all spatial forms" [52].

The American psychologist and behaviorist Skinner had strong implications on enrichment as well. He used operant conditioning to strengthen behavior, created the principles of reinforcement and introduced the process of shaping, techniques that are still used today in many animal training husbandry and medical procedures, and represent a gold standard for dealing with behavioral problems in a variety of settings [50]. He also reported sterile environments causing animals to engage in repetitive behaviors [49]. Hal Markowitz also made significant contributions to the expansion of social consideration about enrichment since the 1970s, being a pioneer in marine mammal research and extending the work by former authors concerning operant conditioning in order to apply this science to improve animal's life [49]. There have been tremendous improvements regarding animal care and captive settings throughout recent years. Replication of wild conditions and stimulation of wild biological repertoires in captive animals have been a long term conservational goal for many zoological institutions. This way, behavioral enrichment programs have become an accepted practice whose most generic priority is addressing and reducing undesirable behaviors [53, 54].

Behavioral enrichment, also known as environmental enrichment, is currently a principle of animal husbandry that has been scientifically proofed to be beneficial [10, 19]. It should be fully incorporated in the daily routine of animals as a tool to maximize their quality of life and discourage undesirable behaviors that emerge as "artifacts of captivity" (e.g., stereotypies) [9, 19]. Enrichment is officially defined as "a dynamic process for enhancing animal environments within the context of the animals' behavioral biology and natural history. Environmental changes are made with the goal of increasing the animals' behavioral choices and drawing out their species-appropriate behaviors, thus enhancing animal welfare" [55]. The aims of behavioral enrichment can be achieved by creating productive environments which encourage each animal to express the natural mental activities and behavioral repertoire of the species, and by adding stimulus that offer complexity and novelty to its routine as well as opportunities that enable it to restore the sense of control it should have over its environment [55]. Behavioral programs have a role in fighting against inactivity and obesity, reducing/eliminating stereotyped and aberrant behavior (e.g., aggression, sexual frustration), and decreasing levels of stress which can, alone, indulge reproduction [9, 55]. For an enrichment program to succeed, it is very important that it is methodically planned in accordance with its objectives and desired outcomes, otherwise it may be more harmful than beneficial [19]. The foundation and logistics of a successful, goal-orientated and self-sustained program can be outlined through AZA reviewed guidelines and protocols so as to represent a master plan from goal setting to re-adjustment, addressing safety issues, providing and keeping up-to-date resources [55]. All animal care staff members and all the professional sectors in the zoological institutions must be involved in the development of an animal enrichment program, as each one plays a critical role in its success [19, 56]. Disney's Animal Kingdom developed the 'S.P.I.D.E.R' framework, a solid model which works as a valuable tool in the development, implementation and maintenance of institutional training and enrichment programs. These programs provide species with appropriate challenges, opportunities and stimulation for all taxa [10, 56]. S.P.I.D.E.R is an acronym for the first letter of each component of the framework [57], as follows: setting goals; planning; implementation; documenting; evaluation; re-adjustment. The last component of the framework actually takes place during all the process of development of an enrichment plan [56]. The goals of a plan are regularly re-adjusted and enrichment activities refined, improved or discontinued to increase effectiveness of a strategy, which may, at some point, be started over again [55]. Five, not mutually exclusive, enrichment categories are generally recognized which will cover the basic needs of an animal and increase a positive utilization of its environment: (1) sensory; (2) structural/physical; (3) social (4) cognitive and (5) food/nutrition [55].

Sensory enrichment refers to the five perceptual senses of sight, smell, hearing, taste and touch [19]. Olfactory stimulation is of the main importance in behavioral enrichment as many species use olfactory signalment to communicate with intra and inter specifics as well as to maintain their territories. They are also driven by their sense of smell to locate prey, reproductive mates or food [54, 58]. Olfactory enrichment may include addition of scented material and both packaged and natural odors [33, 59, 60]. On the other hand, daily removal of natural odors from enclosures through husbandry routine practices should be avoided as it leads to clearance of important olfactory cues in the animal's environment [13]. The value of auditory stimulation to the well-being of animals is still controversial in the literature. It can be vaguely divided into sounds specific of a specie's natural habitat and sounds that are not found in the wild [44]. It is important to bear in mind that the addition of extra noise to environments which can be pretty loud themselves may also have a negative impact in their dwellers, including hearing impairment and communication disconcert between animals [9, 13]. In some cases, the most significant aspect regarding acoustic stimulation so far, may be the overall reduction of the ambient noise [13]. Visual means of enriching the captive environment of animals may include addition of mirrors, moving toys, televisions or other computer-assisted equipment as well as simply allowing the sight of activities outside the enclosure or of a prey [13, 19]. The tactile category includes a varied set of toys, subtracts and other artificial/natural manipulanda, which can be provided in different shapes and textures, either permanently or through a rotation scheme in order to maintain interest, and in close association with the other classes of sensorial enrichment [9, 61].

"**Foraging**", as a concept that comprises searching, retrieving, acquiring and processing food [61], is a time consuming activity that constitutes a major portion of the daily time budget of animals in the wild [19, 62]. Captivity, on the other hand, provides animals with a more limited selection of food types, usually processed diets that are dispensed in highly predicted locations, at fixed feeding times, and in an easily consumed form which does not require natural foraging tactics [9, 62]. Feeding animals through more versatile and natural ways is one of the most widely used enrichment techniques [63].

Structural enrichment highlights the utmost importance of the quality of the space available in overcoming space restrictions [9, 52]. A revolution in zoo enclosure design has led to a proliferation of more naturalistic exhibits which replicate as closely as possible the wild habitat of the species concerned [23, 52]. These exhibits are also functionally evaluated with the priority of creating stimulating and appropriate captive environments according to the specific behaviors and biological needs of each species [55].

Social enrichment involves all forms of social interactions provided direct or indirectly by conspecifics, humans and other species of animals, through physical contact, verbal communication or even olfactory signalment [56]. Many studies instigate the importance of housing appropriate social groupings in the welfare of captive animals [64, 65]. The term "mixed-species exhibits" implies inter-specific associations of animals that would naturally occur in the wild [19].

Cognitive/mental stimulation may be carried out through provision of training sessions, puzzle feeders and other cognitive devices that require animals to solve a problem [19, 55]. Training, based on both classical and operant conditioning principles is a revolutionary way of intellectually challenging the everyday routine of captive animals while managing them to comply with basic husbandry tasks or medical procedures without being forced to do so [61].

Enrichment in its most varied forms elicits investigatory, foraging or marking behavior, social interaction, and creative play. It also provides shade and privacy through hiding places or escape routes, leading to a more efficient use of space [9, 61]. However, the results of every approach will depend on intrinsic factors such as species, age, sex and individual personality [13]. The animal's environment can thus be manipulated and modified in countless ways through a holistic view of the animal's biology, being the limit our own creativity. However, enrichment will not only be beneficial for the animals but for the general public as well. Through promotion of natural species-specific behaviors, enrichment will create valuable and more accurate educational opportunities for the visitors to learn about animal's natural history, biology and conservation. Consequently, it will enhance guest's experiences and their perception of the zoological institutions' mission [19, 55].

4. Conclusion

Veterinarians are irrevocable generalists, which makes them proficient in the holistic approach of disease dynamics. They have not only a broad education in comparative medicine (not a single-species focus) but also in many specialties such as surgery, clinical medicine, anesthesiology, epidemiology, nutrition, pathology, toxicology, theriogenology and behavior. This makes them excellent at understanding both mental and physical needs of an animal, and how well adapted it is to its environment [3, 15]. Wildlife vets are also highly trained in recognizing, diagnosing and understanding disease impact on public health as well as on individuals, populations and whole ecosystems; and, in choosing the most advisable preventive and therapeutic options on a case by case basis [14, 15]. Their ubiquitous knowledge, skills and expertise therefore turns them into valuable key players in planning, implementing and effectively assisting both in-situ and ex-situ conservation projects [2]. As a result, deep collaboration between veterinarians and professionals of other scientific fields such as applied biomedics, epidemiology, ecology, biology and evolutionary genetics, is becoming positively accepted as a new way of integrating health sciences into conservation [2, 15] thus defining Conservation Medicine.

Acknowledgements

The authors wish to thank Dr. Carla Monteiro of the Santo Inácio Zoo, Vila Nova de Gaia, Portugal for her technical and scientific support.

This study was funded by the project UID/CVT/00772/2013 and UID/CVT/00772/2016 supported by the Portuguese Science and Technology Foundation (FCT).

Author details

Diana Raquel Neves Fernandes[1] and Maria de Lurdes Ribeiro Pinto[2]*

1 National Center for the Reproduction of the Iberian Lynx (CNRLI), Herdade das Santinhas, Silves, Portugal

2 Animal and Veterinary Research Centre (CECAV), Trás-os-Montes e Alto Douro University, Vila Real, Portugal

*Address all correspondence to: lpinto@utad.pt

References

[1] Pimm SL, Jenkins CN, Abell R, Brooks TM, Gittleman JL, Joppa LN, et al. The biodiversity of species and their rates of extinction, distribution, and protection. Science. 2014;**344**(6187):1246752. DOI: 10.1126/science.1246752

[2] Deem SL. Conservation medicine to one health: The role of zoologic veterinarians. In: Fowler M, Miller R, editors. Fowler's Zoo and Wild Animal Medicine. 1st ed. Vol. 8. Missouri: Elsevier; 2015. pp. 698-703

[3] Jakob-Hoff R, Warren KS. Conservation medicine for zoo animals. In: Fowler M, Miller R, editors. Fowler's Zoo and Wild Animal Medicine. Vol. 7. Missouri: Elsevier; 2012. pp. 15-23

[4] Karesh W, Cook R. Applications of veterinary medicine to in situ conservation efforts. Oryx. 1995;**29**(4):244-252. DOI: 10.1017/S0030605300021232

[5] Conway W. Wild and zoo animal interactive management and habitat conservation. Biodiversity and Conservation. 1995;**4**:573-594. DOI: 10.1007/BF00222515

[6] Whilde J, Martindale MQ Duffy DJ. Precision wildlife medicine: Applications of the human-centred precision medicine revolution to species conservation. Global Change Biology. 2017;**23**:1792-1805. DOI: 10.1111/gcb.13548

[7] McPhee ME, Carlstead K. Effects of captivity on the behavior of wild mammals. In: Kleiman DG, Allen M, Thompson K, editors. Wild Mammals in Captivity. 2nd ed. Chicago: University of Chicago Press; 2010. pp. 303-313

[8] Broom DM. Coping, stress and welfare. In: Broom DM, editor. Proceedings of Dahlem Conference on Coping with Challenge: Welfare in Animals Including Humans. Berlin: Dahlem University Press; 2001. pp. 1-9

[9] Newberry RC. Environmental enrichment: Increasing the biological relevance of captive environments. Applied Animal Behaviour Science. 1995;**44**:229-243. DOI: 10.1016/0168-1591(95)00616-Z

[10] Mellor DJ, Hunt S, Gusset M, editors. Caring for Wildlife: The World Zoo and Aquarium Animal Welfare Strategy. Gland: WAZA Executive Office; 2015. 87 p

[11] European Association of Zoos and Aquaria (EAZA). Available from: http://www.eaza.net/ [Accessed: Oct 5, 2018]

[12] Broom DM. Animal welfare: Concepts and measurement. Journal of Animal Science. 1991;**69**:4167-4175. DOI: 10.2527/1991.69104167x

[13] Wharton D, Mainka SA. Review: Snow leopard management and husbandry. International Zoo Yearbook. 1997;**35**:139-147. DOI: 10.1111/j.1748-1090.1997.tb01203.x

[14] Deem SL, Karesh WB, Weisman W. Putting theory into practice: Wildlife health in conservation. Conservation Biology. 2001;**15**:1224-1233

[15] Deem SL. Role of the zoo veterinarian in the conservation of captive and free-ranging wildlife. International Zoo Yearbook. 2007;**41**:3-11. DOI: 10.1111/j.1748-1090.2007.00020.x

[16] Minteer BA, Collins JP. Ecological ethics in captivity: Balancing values and responsibilities in zoo and aquarium research under rapid global change. ILAR Journal. 2013;**54**:41-51. DOI: 10.1093/ilar/ilt009

[17] National Geographic [Internet]. 2008. Available from: https://www.nationalgeographic.org/encyclopedia/zoo/ [Accessed: Sep 10, 2018]

[18] Rothfels N. Savages and Beasts: The Birth of the Modern Zoo. Baltimore: Johns Hopkins University Press; 2008. 288 p

[19] Cipreste CF, de Azevedo CS, Young RJ. How to develop a zoo-based environmental enrichment program: Incorporating environmental enrichment into exhibits. In: Kleinman DG, Thompson KV, Baer CK, editors. Wild Mammals in Captivity: Principles and Techniques for Zoo Management. 2nd ed. Chicago: The University of Chicago Press; 2010. pp. 171-180

[20] Moss A, Esson M. The educational claims of zoos: Where do we go from here? Zoo Biology. 2013;**32**:13-18. DOI: 10.1002/zoo.2102

[21] People for the Ethical Treatment of Animals (PETA) [Internet]. 2008. Available from: https://www.peta.org/issues/animals-in-entertainment/zoos-pseudo-sanctuaries/ [Accessed: Sep 20, 2018]

[22] Associations of Zoos and Aquariums [Internet]. 2018. Available from: https://www.aza.org/code-of-ethics [Accessed: Nov 2, 2018]

[23] World Association of Zoos and Aquariums: WAZA [Internet]. 2018. Available from: http://www.waza.org/en/site/home [Accessed: Oct 6, 2018]

[24] Rai S. National Studbook of Snow leopard (*Panthera uncia*). New Delhi: Wildlife Institute of India, Dehradun and Central Zoo Authority; 2015. pp. 20-27

[25] World Health Organization: WHO [Internet]. 2018. Available from: http://www.who.int/about/mission/en/ [Accessed: Oct 5, 2018]

[26] Kreger MD, Hutchins M. Ethics of keeping mammals in zoos and aquariums. In: Kleinman DG, Thompson KV, Baer CK, editors. Wild Mammals in Captivity: Principles and Techniques for Zoo Management. 2nd ed. Chicago: The University of Chicago Press; 2010. pp. 3-10

[27] Mikota SK, Aguilar RF. Management protocols for animal in captive propagation and reintroduction programmes. Revue Scientifique et Technique (International Office of Epizootics). 1996;**15**:191-208

[28] Conway W. The practical difficulties and financial implications of endangered species breeding programmes. International Zoo Yearbook. 1986;**24/25**:210-219

[29] Bloomqvist L. The captive snow leopard in 2007. In: International Pedigree Book for Snow Leopards, *Uncia uncia*. Helsinki: Helsinki Zoo; 2008. 175 p

[30] Jackson RM, Mishra C, McCarthy TM, Ale SB. Snow leopards: Conflict and conservation. In: Macdonald DW, Andrew J, editors. The Biology and Conservation of Wild Felids. Oxford: Oxford University Press; 2010. pp. 417-430

[31] Kagan R, Veasey J. Challenges of zoo animal welfare. In: Kleinman DG, Thompson KV, Baer CK, editors. Wild Mammals in Captivity: Principles and Techniques for Zoo Management. 2nd ed. Chicago: The University of Chicago Press; 2010. pp. 11-21

[32] Hosey GR, Melfi VA, Pankhurst SJP. Zoo Animals: Behaviour, Management and Welfare. Vol. 643. Oxford: Oxford University Press; 2009

[33] McGlone JJ, Anderson DL. Synthetic maternal pheromone stimulates feeding behaviour and weight gain in pigs. Journal of Animal Science. 2008;**80**:3179-3183

[34] Brambell Report. Report of the Technical Committee to Enquire Into The welfare of Animals Kept under Intensive Livestock Husbandry Systems [Internet]. London, UK: Her Majesty's Stationery Office. 1965. Available from: http://edepot.wur.nl/134379 [Accessed: Nov 3, 2018]

[35] The National Archives [Internet]. 2018. Available from: http://webarchive.nationalarchives.gov.uk/20121003015231/http://www.defra.gov.uk/fawc/about/five-freedoms/ [Accessed: Nov 2, 2018]

[36] Webster J. Animal Welfare: A Cool Eye Towards Eden. Wiley; 1995. 284 p

[37] Kolter L, Zander R. Potential and limitations of environmental enrichment in managing behavioural problems of polar beras. In: Proceedings of the Second International Conference on Environmnetal Enrichment; 21-25 August 1995; Copenhagen: Copenhagen Zoo; 1995. p.131-141

[38] World Organization for Animal Health (OIE). Terrestrial Animal Health Code. 20th ed. Paris: World Organisation for Animal Health (OIE); 2011. pp. 289-382

[39] Broom DM. Indicators of poor welfare. British Veterinary Journal. 1986;**142**:524-526

[40] Melfi VA. There are big gaps in our knowledge, and thus approach, to zoo animal welfare: A case for evidence-based zoo animal management. Zoo Biology. 2009;**28**:574-588. DOI: 10.1002/zoo.20288

[41] Boissy A, Manteuffel G, Jensen MB, Moe RO, Spruijt B, Keeling LJ, et al. Assessment of positive emotions in animals to improve their welfare. Physiology & Behavior. 2007;**92**:375-397. DOI: 10.1016/j.physbeh.2007.02.003

[42] Webster AJF. Farm animal welfare: The five freedoms and the free market. The Veterinary Journal. 2001;**161**:229-237. DOI: 10.1053/tvjl.2000.0563

[43] Dawkins MS. Using behaviour to assess animal welfare. Animal Welfare. 2004;**13**:S3-S7

[44] European Comission [Internet]. 2018. Available from: https://ec.europa.eu/food/animals/welfare_en [Accessed: Sep 27, 2018]

[45] Broom DM. The scientific assessment of animal welfare. Applied Animal Behaviour Science. 1988;**20**:5-19

[46] Rees PA. Studying Captive Animals: A Workbook of Methods in Behaviour, Welfare and Ecology. Oxford: Wiley; 2015. 318 p

[47] Skinner BF. The Behavior of Organisms. Cambridge: Copley Publishing Groups; 1938. 473 p

[48] Bishop J, Hosey G, Plowman A, editors. Handbook of Zoo Research, Guidelines for Conducting Research in Zoos. London: BIAZA; 2013. pp. 63-71

[49] Cambridge Center for Behavioral Studies [Internet]. 2018. Available from: https://behavior.org/help-centers/animal-behavior/enrichment/

[50] B.F. Skinner Foundation [Internet]. 2018. Available from: http://www.bfskinner.org/ [Accessed: Oct 10, 2018]

[51] Maple TL. Prof. Dr. Heini Hediger (1908-1992). Zoo Biology. 1992;**11**:369-372

[52] Hediger H. Man and Animal in the Zoo: Zoo Biology. New York: Delacorte Press; 1969. 303 p

[53] Mason GJ, Latham NR. Can't stop, won't stop: Is stereotypy a reliable animal welfare indicator? Animal Welfare. 2004;**13**:S57-S69

[54] Skibiel AL, Trevino HS, Naugher K. Comparison of several types of enrichment for captive felids. Zoo Biology. 2007;**26**:371-381. DOI: 10.1002/zoo.20147

[55] Young RJ. Environmental enrichment for captive animals. Oxford: Blackwell Science. 2003. 228 p

[56] Animal Enrichment [Internet]. 2018. Available from: http://www.animalenrichment.org/spider

[57] Sevenich MM, Mellen J. Animal Training: [Internet]. 2018. Available from: http://www.animaltraining.org/spider/ [Accessed: Oct 13, 2018]

[58] Hurst JL, Beynon RJ, Roberts SC, Wyatt TD. Chemical Signals in Vertebrates. New York: Springer; 2008. 417 p

[59] Estelles MG, Mills DS. Signs of travel-related problems in dogs and their response to treatment with dog-appeasing pheromone. Veterinary Record. 2006;**59**(5): 143-148

[60] Graham L, Wells DL, Hepper PG. The influence of olfactory stimulation on the behaviour of dogs housed in a rescue shelter. Apllied Animal Behaviour Science. 2005;**91**:143-153

[61] Tresz H. Contra freeloading (working for food) at the Phoenix zoo. ABMA Wellspring. 2010;**11**:8-21

[62] Newberry RC. The space-time continuum, and its relevance for farm animals. Etologia. 1993;**3**:219-234

[63] Young RJ. The importance of food presentation for animal welfare and conservation. Proceedings of the Nutrition Society. 1997;**56**:1095-1104

[64] Shepherdson DJ. Environmental enrichment: Past, present and future. International Zoo Yearbook. 2003;**38**:118-124

[65] Price EE, Stoinski TS. Group size: Determinants in the wild and implications for the captive housing of wild mammals in zoos. Applied Animal Behaviour Science. 2007;**10**:255-264. DOI: 10.1016/j.applanim.2006.05.021

Chapter 8

Reptilian Skin and Its Special Histological Structures

Catrin Sian Rutland, Pia Cigler and Valentina Kubale

Abstract

Reptilian skin is covered with scales forming armor that makes it watertight and enables reptiles to live on land in contrast to amphibians. An important part of the skin is the horny epidermis, with thick *stratum corneum* in which waxes are arranged in membrane-like layers. In lizards and snakes, the whole skin is covered in overlapping epidermal scales and in turtles and crocodiles in dermal scutes. The cornified part of the epidermis is strengthened by β-keratin and sometimes α-keratin. In crocodiles and many turtles, the outer scale surface consists of β-keratin and the hinge region containing α-keratin. In lizards and snakes, both keratins form continuous layers with the α-keratin below the β-keratin. Some reptiles have developed a sensitive mechanosensory system in the skin. The colors of reptile skin are produced by melanocytes and three types of chromatophores: melanophores, xanthophores, and iridophores. The color patterns may be fixed or the chromatophores may provide rapid color change. Skin from different species of reptiles, turtles (red-eared slider (*Trachemys scripta elegans*)), snakes (Emerald tree boa (*Corallus caninus*) and Burmese python (*Python bivittatus*)), Cuvier's dwarf caiman (*Paleosuchus palpebrosus*), lizards (Leopard Gecko (*Eublepharis macularius*)), and Green iguana (*Iguana iguana*), were examined with histology techniques and compared.

Keywords: skin, histology, reptiles, special features

1. Reptiles

Reptiles are one of the six main animal groups together with amphibians, invertebrates, fish, birds, and mammals. They are tetrapods that diverged from ancestral amphibians approximately 340 million years ago. There are two characteristics that early reptiles had developed when diverging from amphibians: scales and amniotic eggs (eggs with an internal fluid membrane), which are still of great importance for them. Extant reptiles are represented by four orders: Squamata (lizards, snakes and worm-lizards), Crocodilia (alligators and crocodiles), Chelonia (tortoises and turtles), and Rhynchocephalia (tuatara) [1]. Squamates are the most diverse from all of the groups and have exceptional skull mobility. The only exception to this exceptional skull mobility is the almost extinct tuatara, which only lives on a few New Zealand islands. This reptile has a skull which is not joined, the reptiles grow slowly and reproduce at a slow rate and have a prominent parietal eye on top of the head.

Snakes are carnivorous reptiles with highly mobile jaws, which enable them to swallow prey much larger than they are. They are legless (some species retain a pelvic girdle) and have an elongated body, this means that paired organs appear one in front of other and they only have one functional lung. Some species have venom, used primarily to kill prey. Their skin is covered in scales and snakes are not slimy [2]. Lizards are quadrupedal squamates, except some legless, snake-like-bodied species. Often, they are territorial and have many antipredator strategies, such as camouflage, venom, reflex bleeding, and the ability to destroy and then regenerate their tails after destruction. They are covered in overlapping keratin scales, enabling them to live in the driest deserts on the earth [3, 4].

Crocodilians are the largest reptiles, and include the alligators, crocodiles, gharials, and caimans. They have elongated, structurally reinforced skulls, powerful jaw muscles, teeth in sockets, and a complete secondary palate; they are oviparous and, interestingly, adults provide extensive parental care to young.

Turtles are among the most ancient of the reptiles alive today and have changed little since they first appeared 200 million years ago. They have a protective shell that encloses their body and provides protection and camouflage. They have keratinized plates instead of teeth and a shell that consists of a carapace and plastron [5, 6].

2. Histology of reptile's skin

An integumental challenge for reptilian's terrestrial life was developing mechanisms in order to prevent water loss and to protect against ultraviolet irradiation, mechanical shields which offered protection and enabled evolution of different types of reptilian scales and scutes [3, 7].

Some skin histology features are similar between mammals and reptiles; on the other hand, they also have numerous differences. Reptiles have a reputation that they are "slimy" when we touch and hold them; however, they have dry skin, which has even fewer glands than mammals or amphibians. The main special feature of their skin is that the **epidermis** is heavily keratinized with a layer, which also prevents water loss. This feature reflects their greater commitment to a terrestrial existence. Scales are present but are fundamentally different from the dermal scales of fish. In reptiles, scales cannot be scraped off as in fish because they are an integral part of the skin. The reptilian scale usually lacks the bony under support of any significant structural contribution from dermis. It is a fold in the surface epidermis, an epidermal scale. The junction between adjacent epidermal scales provides a flexible hinge. If the epidermal scale is large and plate-like, it is also termed scutes. Epidermal scales in different species can be overgrown and skin protrusions can be formed in different regions, such as microornamentation, pits, sensory receptors, spines, horn-like processes, crests, scutes, plastron, carapace, and some others [7, 8]. These protrusions are essentially only of epidermal origin, without dermal participation [1]. In the perfect resting phase, the epidermis generally consists of four layers of dead but fully differentiated keratinocytes and basal live keratinocyte layer that form three main layers: *stratum basale (germinativum)*, *stratum granulosum,* and *stratum corneum*.

The inner layer, *stratum germinativum*, consists of cuboidal dividing cells that produce the protein keratin. The intermediate layer (*stratum granulosum*) has a lipid-rich film that plays a major role in providing water-permeable barrier in the skin. The outer *stratum corneum* is heavily keratinized in scales. Two forms of keratin are produced in reptiles: α-keratin, which is flexible, and β-keratin, which provides strength and hardness and is unique to reptiles. β-keratin is found on the chelonian shells, whereas α-keratin is found in the hinges or between the scutes [9–11]. It is in these weaker links that mites or infections can be present. The thick, keratinized skin of reptiles is at the expense of the cutaneous sensation. Reptiles have far less sensory feeling in their skin than birds or mammals, which is why they are more at risk from thermal burns in captivity (e.g., lizards and hot stones). In many reptiles, dermal bones (*gastralia*) are present especially in the abdominal area; however, they are not associated with scales.

The main layers of epidermis change prior to molting in the reptiles that slough large pieces of the cornified skin layer. In the turtles and crocodiles, sloughing of skin is modest, comparable to birds and mammals, in whom small flakes fall off at irregular intervals. But in lizards, and especially in snakes, shedding of the cornified layer, termed molting or ecdysis, results in removal of extensive sections of superficial epidermis. As molting begins, the *stratum basale*, which has given rise to the *strata granulosum* (inner) and *corneum* (outer), duplicates the deeper layers of granulosum and corneum, pushing up under the old layers. White blood cells invade the *stratum intermedium*, a temporary layer between old and new skin. These white blood cells are thought to promote the separation and loss of the old superficial layer of the skin [8]. Molting of different reptile species will be discussed in more detail later in the chapter.

The **dermis** in reptiles consists of fibrous connective tissue, blood and lymphatic vessels, nerves, and pigmentary cells. At the areas where dermal bones support the epidermis, bony plates called osteoderms, plates of dermal bone, are located under epidermal scales. They are present in crocodilians, some lizards, and some extinct species. Some bones of the turtle shell are modified osteoderms which have fused with the vertebrae to form a shell.

Subcutaneous layer (*hypodermis*, hypoderm, and *subcutis*) is the layer of tissue, which lies beneath dermis and mainly consists of fibroblasts, adipose cells, and macrophages. Subcutaneous fat is mostly poorly developed in reptiles in comparison to mammals. Some species are known for substantial subcutaneous fat pads, such as some species of geckos like the Mediterranean house gecko (*Hemidactylus turcicus*), and some of the snakes and lizards have paired abdominal "fat bodies" (*corpora adiposa*) that serve as the primary location for fat storage in adipose tissue. Also, the tail, especially in geckos, can be a large deposit of the subcutaneous tissue, however not in the snakes. These tail deposits include "inner fat" surrounding the caudal vertebrae, as well as subcutaneous caudal fat and are most concentrated near the base of a tail. These fat tissues could be for some animals the major adipose store in the body [12, 13].

Integumental glands of reptiles are usually restricted to certain areas of the body. In different species, there are some glandular-type tissues in different parts of the body, such as rows of femoral glands under femoral pores alongside the inner part of the thigh region of the hindlimb, which are observed especially in males. In some species of Crocodilians and turtles, scent glands are present. In male and female alligators, one pair of scent glands open in cloaca and another pair on the margins of the lower jaw. In some turtles, scent glands can produce quite pungent odors, especially when the animal is alarmed by handling. Precloacal pores are observed in some lizards and crocodiles. Most integumental glands in reptiles are thought to play a role in reproductive behavior or when predators are close, and their social role has not yet been well studied [8, 9, 11].

3. Reptile groups and their special skin features, especially their scales/scutes

The skin of reptiles reflects their greater commitment to a terrestrial existence as mentioned earlier in the chapter. Keratinization is extensive and skin glands are fewer than in amphibians. Scales are present, but these are fundamentally different from the dermal scales of fish. The reptilian scale usually lacks the bony under support or any significant structural contribution from the dermis. Instead, it is a fold in the surface epidermis, hence, an epidermal scale. The junction between adjacent epidermal scales is the flexible hinge (**Figure 1**). If the epidermal scale is large and

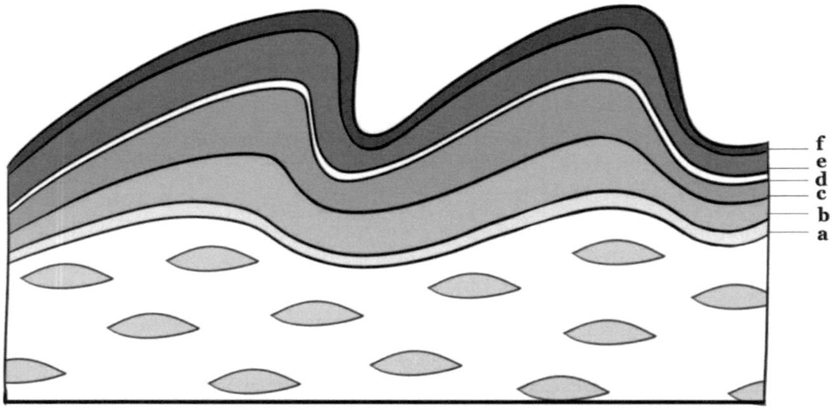

Figure 1.
Layers of epidermis in reptile skin, consisting of stratum basale (germinal layer) (b), where we find a layer of live cells, and then dead but fully differentiated layers of keratinocytes, which are also named α-layer (c), mesos layer (d), β-layer (e) and Oberhäutchen layer (f). Germinal layer lies on the basal lamina (a) and below lies the tissue of the dermis. Fully differentiated layers are parts of stratum granulosum (intermedial layer) with a stratum corneum, consisting of α-keratin and β-keratin. The junction between epidermal scales is the flexible hinge (adopted from Chang et al. [1] and designed by Pia Cigler).

plate-like, it is sometimes termed a scute. Additionally, epidermal scales may be modified into crests, spines, or horn-like processes. Although not usually associated with scales, dermal bone is present in many reptiles. The gastralia, a collection of bones in the abdominal area, are examples of these. Where dermal bones support the epidermis, they are called osteoderms, plates of dermal bone located under the epidermal scales. Osteoderms are found in Crocodilians, some lizards, and some extinct reptiles. Some bones of the turtle shell are probably modified osteoderms.

Scales have many important functions, such as playing vital roles in skin permeability and providing protection from abrasion, and therefore tend to be thicker dorsally than ventrally. In some species, they form into large plates and shields on the head. In snakes, they are widened ventrally to form gastropeges, which are important for locomotion [1, 8].

3.1 Lizards and their skin properties

3.1.1 Scales

The lizard's skin is specific due to scales that form dense tight rows. Lizard scales vary in form from tubercular to plate-like or even largely overlapping each other in formation. The scales originate from the epidermal superficial layer of the skin and form keratinized wrinkles and may have bony plates underlying them (*osteoderms*). They are very close to each other, and links between them allow them to move in all directions. In lizards, scales can vary in form and be modified into crests, spikes, or horns, depending on the type of lizard and on the body part of the lizard and are often of use in taxonomically differentiating species. On the head and on the ventral part, scales are plate-shaped. Scales are important to prevent water loss from the body, as well as to protect the body from injury, because the lizards touch the ground with the ventral surface of the body and thus damage the skin. The skin in the lizard does not follow the growth of the body, so they have to change it, which does not happen in one piece but in several smaller pieces [14].

In some lizards, it is characteristic that their fingers are covered with large scales. These scales serve them to move easier as in the case of the basilisk lizard (*Basiliscus*

basiliscus), especially on the water surface or are helpful in the sand skink (*Neoseps reynoldsi*) to move in the sand. Geckos (Gekkonidae) have flattened fingers, characterized by around 20 leaf-like formations on the ventral side of the toes, named lamellas, with a structure that enables animals to climb on the vertical and very smooth surfaces (**Figure 2**). Lamellas consist of seatae (110 μm in length and 4.2μm in width), which are similarly oriented and uniformly distributed in arrays [14]. Each seta branches to form a nanoarray of hundreds of spatular structures, which are 0.2 μm in length and width at the tip which then make adjacent contact with the surface. Gecko setae are formed primarily of β-keratin with some α-keratin components [15].

The skin glands are mostly restricted to certain parts of the body. Thus, in the medial side of the thighs of many lizards, for example, Green Iguana (*Iguana iguana*), there are femoral pores, beneath which femoral glands are located. These glands are larger and usually more developed in males. They secrete a waxed secretion that contains various pheromones relevant to the mating period or when the animal feels endangered. They also help to determine sex in these species [14].

The lizards do not have an external ear; however, in some species, they have a fold of the skin and tympanic membrane that can be seen from the side on the head in a shallow recess. This membrane is covered by a thin membrane in some species that is also changed in the process of ecdysis.

Some lizards such as Green Iguana (*Iguana iguana*) have partial third eye. This organ is a superficial parietal gland which also contains a lens, cornea, and retina, and is located immediately below the skin in the parietal opening between the parietal and frontal bones. The partial eye is a cavitary organ, which is constructed from epithelial cells that contain secretion glands and photoreceptors that convert light stimuli into neuroendocrine messages that can play an important role in thermoregulation but also in hormone production [16].

Lizard skin contains classical skin layers, which can vary in morphology at different positions. Here, we compare skin of the Leopard Gecko (*Eublepharis macularius*) (**Figure 3**) with the skin of the Green Iguana (*Iguana iguana*) (**Figure 4**), both sampled from the dorsal region. The most visible difference in the epidermis was seen in the level of keratinization, where the skin of the Green Iguana was keratinized to a higher extent and the outermost β-layer was much more pronounced. The second most prominent feature observed are the melanocytes, where in the Green Iguana the melanocytes are hardly seen at all. On the other hand, Leopard Geckos can vary very much in color and they exist in various color mutations

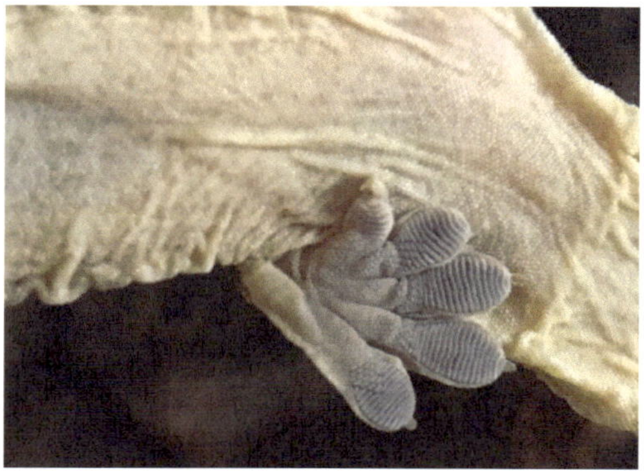

Figure 2.
The ventral view of a New Caledonian Giant Gecko (Rhacodactylus leachianus) climbing a vertical glass surface. On the ventral view of the foot of a New Caledonian Giant Gecko, a foot adhesive system is observed with adhesive lamellas which consist of microscale array of setae, which are together clustered in tetrads (Photography, Valentina Kubale).

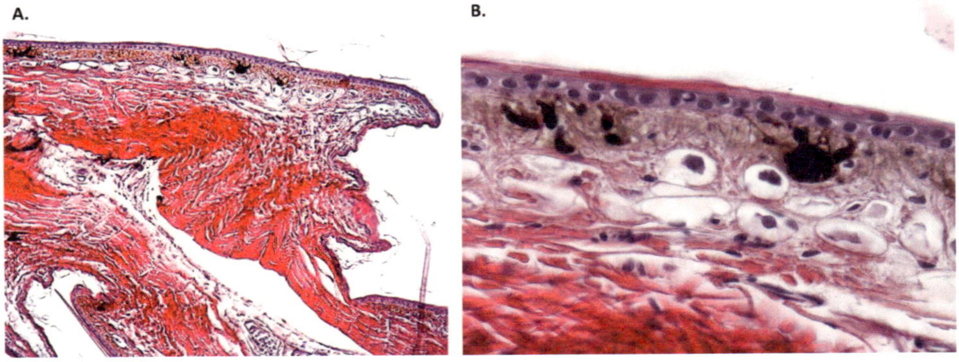

Figure 3.
Dorsum skin histology of the Leopard Gecko (Eublepharis macularius) by H&E staining. The sample was taken in the resting stage of the epidermis, when the animal was not in the process of ecdysis. In epidermis, the most visible part is the basal layer with keratinocytes with nuclei, which are dividing by mitosis. In the figure is the part with overlapping scale. The cornified α-layer is very well visible. The intervening mature stratum (mesos) consists of a few layers of cells, which are often not very well seen under this magnification. Partially is also separated from the lower strata as well as the outermost β-layer. In the dermis, fibrous connective tissue, vessels, nerves, melanophores, and Merkel mechanoreceptor cells are observed. (A) 100× magnification, (B) 400× magnification.

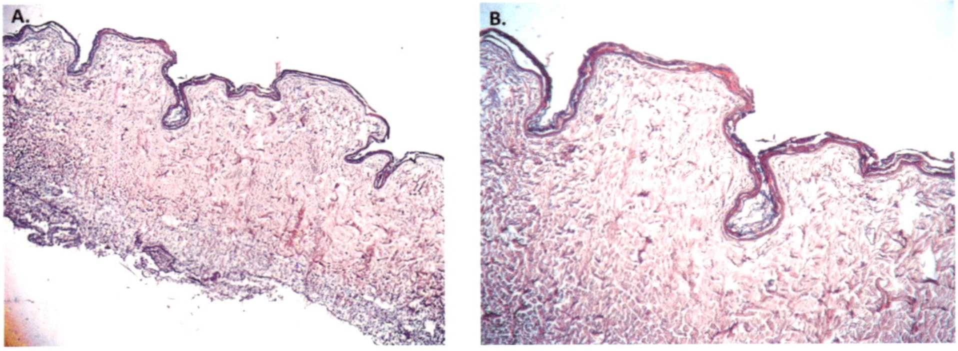

Figure 4 .
Dorsum skin histology of the Green Iguana (Iguana iguana) by H&E staining. The sample was taken in the resting stage of the epidermis, when the animal was not in the process of ecdysis. In epidermis, different layers are observed. The stratum granulosum is not very clearly distinguishable with the nuclei. Cornified α-layer and the outermost β-layer are very visible. In the dermis, fibrous connective tissue, vessels, and nerves are observed. Fibers of the connective tissue are laid in a kind of pattern (A) 100× magnification, (B) 200× magnification.

(termed morphs). Our sample originates from the most common one, which is basic yellow in color with black spots, which also contains more melanophores. Other morphs include the high yellow (less black spots), hypomelanistic with ten or less dark spots on the body or on the other hand hypermelanistic, which has darker pigmentation but is not black in color. Blizzards are morphs that are completely pattern less. The lavender Gecko has light violet or lavender color included, the tangerine one has an orange color included in its coloration, the carrot tail has orange color on the tail and there are some more variations in color also present in different geckos [14].

3.1.2 The production of color

Especially important for camouflage (mimicry) is the skin color. Skin color is susceptible to changes depending on the amount of sunlight and it may be darker or lighter. Chromatophores are pigment-containing cells found in the dermis of the skin and provide a large range of colors by changing the position of their granules. This ability is particularly significant for the chameleons, although it is also observed to a lesser extent in other types of lizards, such as the New Caledonian Giant Gecko (**Figure 5**), and in some species when light and temperature influence change of skin color to more pronounced such as in the Saharan Uromastyx (*Uromastyx geyri*) (**Figure 6**). The color of the lizard's skin can also be affected by the environment and by the endocrine system [17, 18]. These pigment cells are not just confined to skin but can also occur in the peritoneum of some species, for example in turtles. Animals of the same species during breeding may, due to different mutations, change their basic color and thus produce offspring with new patterns, which are new morphs.

Chameleons are an extreme example group of lizards, and, of all the reptiles, they have the highest ability in relation to changing their skin coloration and pattern through combinations of pink, blue, red, orange, green, black, brown, light blue, yellow, turquoise, and purple [19]. Chameleons change skin color depending on the temperature of the surrounding area, their physical condition, intraspecies signaling and communication. Color change is also important for their camouflage. It signals a chameleon's physiological condition and also shows its intentions toward other chameleons [19]. Chameleons tend to show brighter colors when displaying aggression to other chameleons, and darker colors when they signal they are not fighting [20].

Chameleons transform color by changing the space between the guanine crystals which are present in specialized cells named chromatophores. The color change is based upon the wavelength of light reflected off of the crystals. The skin of the chameleons is as in other reptiles consisting of epidermis, dermis, and hypodermis. The important features chameleons have regarding skin color are located in the dermis. It is within the dermis that the blood vessels, nerves, skin muscles, and special cells named chromatophores are present. The chromatophores contain guanine crystals and are subdivided into differing types including iridophores, xanthophores, erythrophores, guanophores, and melanophores (**Figure 7**).

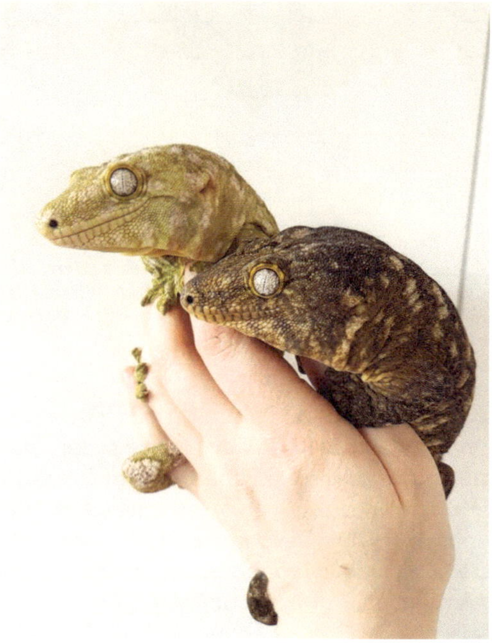

Figure 5.
Different color of the skin in the New Caledonian Giant Gecko caused by environment (Rhacodactylus leachianus) in the same species (Photography, Pia Cigler).

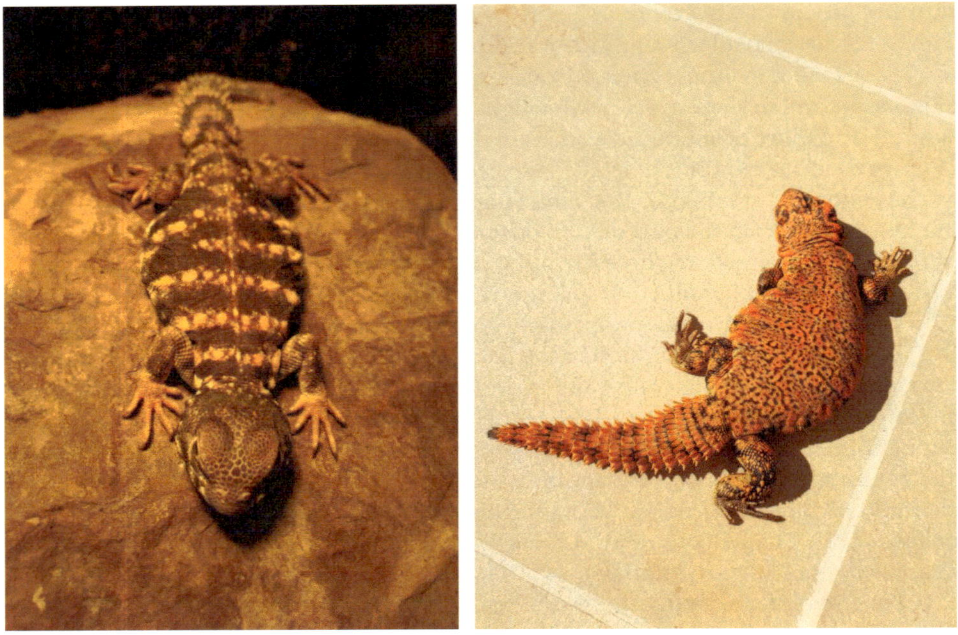

Figure 6 .
Different color of the skin in the Saharan Uromastyx (Uromastyx geyri) influenced by temperature and sunlight (Photography, Pia Cigler).

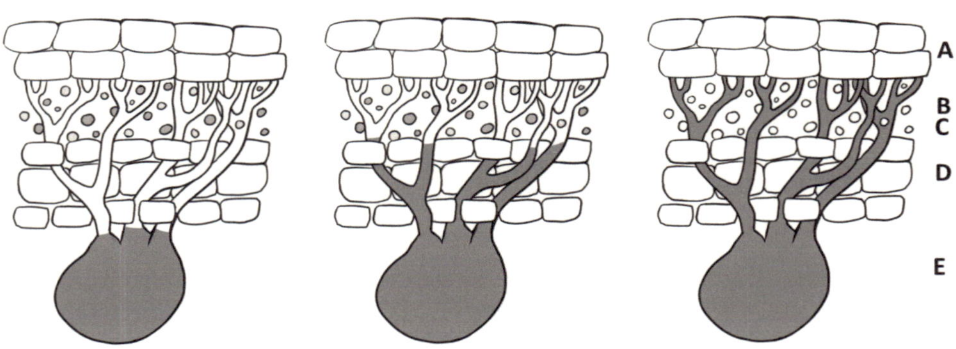

Figure 7.
Chromatophores in reptiles (Chameleons) (adapted from Krey and Farayalah [21] and designed by Pia Cigler). Different chromatophores lie in the different layers of the epidermis and dermis. A. Keratin layer, B. Xanthophores, C. Erythrophores, D. Guanophores, E. Melanophores. The three figures show how coloration is achieved through their extensions.

The iridophores (granulophores) lie in the dermis. They are the most important for true color change, not just changing shades of the same color. They contain semi-crystalline nanocrystals of the amino acid guanine (the breakdown of uric acid) that reflects light. They are arranged in a network in a surface and in a deeper layer. In the deeper layer, iridophore crystals have a protective role for the organism against harmful rays. At the surface of the iridophore, smaller crystals are located, which can diffract different wavelengths of light, depending on their arrangement and density. The blue wavelengths are reflected more to produce a blue coloration in an effect called Tyndall scattering. When combined with the yellow carotenoids, they emit green color, which is a common camouflage in many reptiles [9]. Guanophores contain a colorless crystalline substance called guanin and reflect among others the blue part of light. Xanthophores produce the pigments called pteridines and are important for yellow shades of the skin. Erythrophores contain the pigment carotene, which they get from the other parts of the body and are important for shades of red. Both types of cells are located above the iridophores and when they cover each other they can form different color combinations. Green color is the consequence of the yellow pigment which covers the refracted blue color coming from iridophores. Melanophores produce the pigment melanin and they lie the deepest within the dermis. Pigment melanin-containing cells give rise to black, brown, yellow, and gray coloration. Albinism in reptiles is caused by lack of melanin. The carotenoid cells are found beneath the epidermis above the melanophores and produce yellow, red, and orange pigments [9], so albino reptiles are often yellow to orange color.

Dispersion of the pigment-containing organelles is only a partial mechanism [17]. Different chromatophores are arranged in two superimposed layers within their skin that control their color and thermoregulation. The top layer contains a lattice of guanine nanocrystals, and by exciting this lattice, the spacing between the nanocrystals can be manipulated, which in turn affects which wavelengths of light are reflected and which are absorbed. Exciting the lattice increases the distance between the nanocrystals, and the skin reflects longer wavelengths of light. Thus, in a relaxed state, the crystals reflect blue and green, but in an excited state, the longer wavelengths such as yellow, orange, green, and red are reflected [14, 20].

4. Snake's skin and scale features

In snakes, the skin is entirely covered with scales, specific to reptiles. The scales are set together as piles covering each other and are comprised of the upper part of mucosal layer of the skin with subcutaneous tissue below; they are keratinized and protect snakes from skin injuries and dehydration, basically to make it air-proof. When considering the position on the body, they have a different layout and shape. Scales, especially on the head, have an important role in determining the species of snakes. Smaller scales are found dorsally on the body and are placed in several rows. On the ventral, abdominal part of the body, scales are wide and transversally positioned. The shape and number of scales on the head, back, and belly are characteristic to each family, genus, and species. Scales have a nomenclature analogous to the position on the body. In "advanced" (Caenophidian) snakes, the broad belly scales and rows of dorsal scales correspond to the vertebrae, allowing scientists to count the vertebrae without dissection [14].

Scales protect the body of the snake, aid it in locomotion, allow moisture to be retained within and give simple or complex coloration patterns which help in camouflage and antipredator display. In some snakes, scales have been modified over time to serve other functions such as those of "'eyelash" fringes, and the most distinctive modification—the *rattle* of the North American rattlesnakes. The snakes also use scales for different types of movement because they have lost their limbs through the evolution process [22].

With the abdominal part of their scales, snakes can resist the unevenness of the surface and move across bare terrain such as sand and roads, where they cannot push off rocks and branches (lateral undulation type of movement) and with their muscle strength push their body forward. Besides that, it is mathematically proven that snakes also rely on the frictional properties of their scales to slide [23].

The resistance of a snake's belly scales is highest when its body is sliding sideways, rather than forward or backward. Snakes also seem to lift the parts of their bodies where friction is slowing movement the most, enabling them to slither faster. Snakes can move by folding themselves into pleats, contracting their bellies, contorting into helices or slithering in an S-shape. Scientists suggested that the snakes' belly scales, which can catch small bumps in the ground, might also aid movement. Behind the cloaca, scales are smaller and usually positioned in two lines. When closely observed, the border between the body and the tail is seen [23].

Snakes have pigmented scales; their color can change in certain species and some snakes are also albino snakes. Color of a young snake can be brighter than in adults and may also depend on the geographical position of the snake. In the cubs of green tree python (*Morelia viridis*), the color is yellowish to orange, however adult animals become green. The color of some boa species is also associated with the period of the day, where they are mostly darker at daylight and brighter at night time.

There is a polymorphism in snakes, but it is not common. It can be seen, for example, in the Turks Island Boa (*Epicrates chrysogaster*) and the Californian Royal Snake (*Lampropeltis getula californiae*), in which cells at the part of the snake may appear on individual animals forming a pattern and on the other part forming lines at the same time. During breeding of snakes, genetic mutations have emerged recently, and partial albinos are possible. During breeding, due to various mutations in the Ball Python (*Python regius*), color change may occur, and new species of morphs can be developed (**Figure 8**).

Snake skin contains pigmented cells and snakes use their color to camouflage (mimicry) or in order to give warning signs. A special form of mimicry is imitation of color, in which poor poisonous and non-lethal species of snake, such as the Arizona Mountain Kingsnake (*Lampropeltis pyromelana pyromelana*) (**Figure 9**), mimics an extremely poisonous painted coral snake (*Micrurus corallinus*) to protect themselves from predators [14].

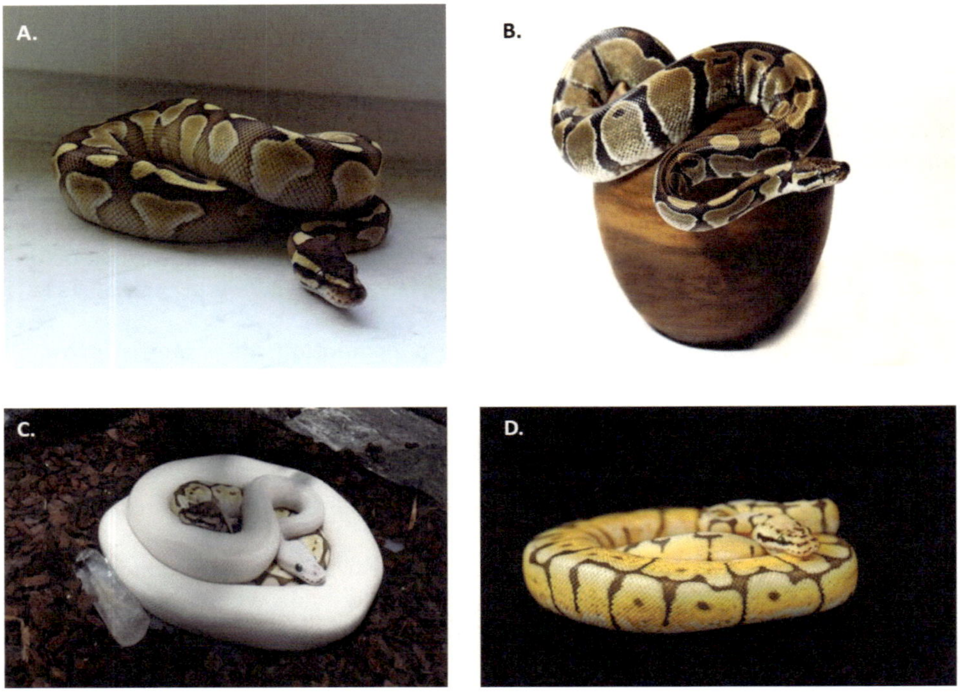

Figure 8.
A portrait of different patterns, colors, and morphs of Ball python (Python regius) (Photography, Leja Hrovatin, Nina Bajec, Nika Glavina, and Tilen Holynski). Very well-known and desired morphs are: Super Pastel Ivory morph (C), Piebald morph, Super Pastel Axanthic; Butter Pastel: Cinnamon, lesser (A), Super Pastel Spider, (D) Coral Glow/Banana in the comparison to normal ball python (B).

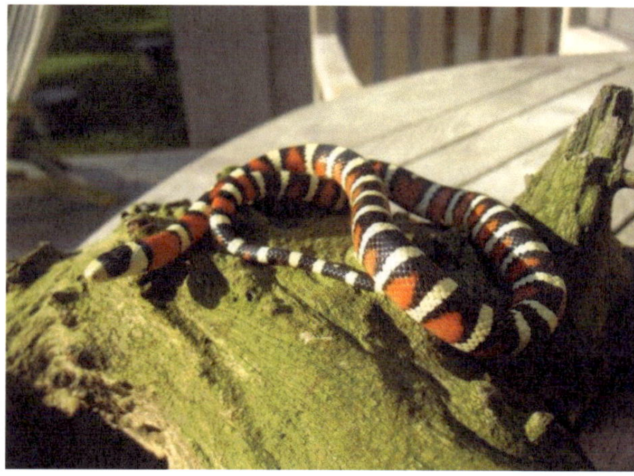

Figure 9.
Arizona Mountain Kingsnake (Lampropeltis pyromelana pyromelana) (Photography Pia Cigler).

Snake's skin is similarly as in lizard's consisted of germinal layer of the epidermis spinosus-like keratinocytes that alternate to hard (β) and soft (α) layers. Samples from two different species of snakes were observed histologically and skin samples were collected from different parts of the body. We have observed skin at the abdominal (ventral) part and the tail of the Burmese Python (*Python bivittatus*) (**Figure 10**) and the lip part of the Emerald Tree Boa (*Corallus caninus*) (**Figure 11**). From the outer scale surface toward the dermis are the *oberhautchen* layer, β-layer, mesos layer, α-layer, lacunar layer, and the clear layer [1, 24, 25].

Iridescence is caused by the physical properties of light on the thin and transparent outer layer of the skin. When light strikes from an angle, the light spectrum is split into wavelengths of different colors. Depending on the color of the scales, this will cause iridescent effect when the snake moves. This feature is more obvious in black or dark snakes like the white-lipped python (*Liasis albertisii*) (**Figure 12**) [14].

Snakes living among the leaves are most often green, and those living in the desert are often yellowish or reddish. Snakes have no skin glands other than cloacal glands. Some species can detect infrared light. Primitive boas have pronounced sensory receptors in the skin and can detect mice at a distance of 15 cm. Between the nostrils and the eye, in some snakes, there are special infrared receptors (pits) that allow them to feel hot-blooded animals and to attack them in the dark. These receptors are innerved with *n. mandibularis*, *n. maxillaris,* and *n. ophthalmicus* (branch of *n. trigeminus*). Along the upper and lower lumbar scales, there are fewer pits, which are also innervated by the branches of *n. trigeminus*. These organs are extremely sensitive to temperature changes of as much as 0.002°C [14].

At the ends of the tails of rattlesnakes (*Crotalus sp.*), there is a special anatomical adjustment—a rattle. Also, their name derives from the Greek word *krótalon*, which means "rattle" or "castanet," and refers to the rattle on the end of the tail which makes this group (genera *Crotalus* and *Sistrurus*) very distinctive [26]. The rattle consists of up to 20 loosely interlocking hollow shells, each of which is at one point the scale covering the tip of the tail. Their number depends on the type and gender of the animal. In most other snakes, the tail tip is cone-shaped and not much thicker than the rest of the skin. It is shed along with the rest of molt. However, in rattlesnakes, it does not shed, and it also gets elongated, since younger specimens may shed three to four times per year, every time adding a new segment to the rattle. The end of the tail is much thicker and round shaped at the end, with one or two annular constrictions to prevent it from falling off. Before each shedding, a new button will

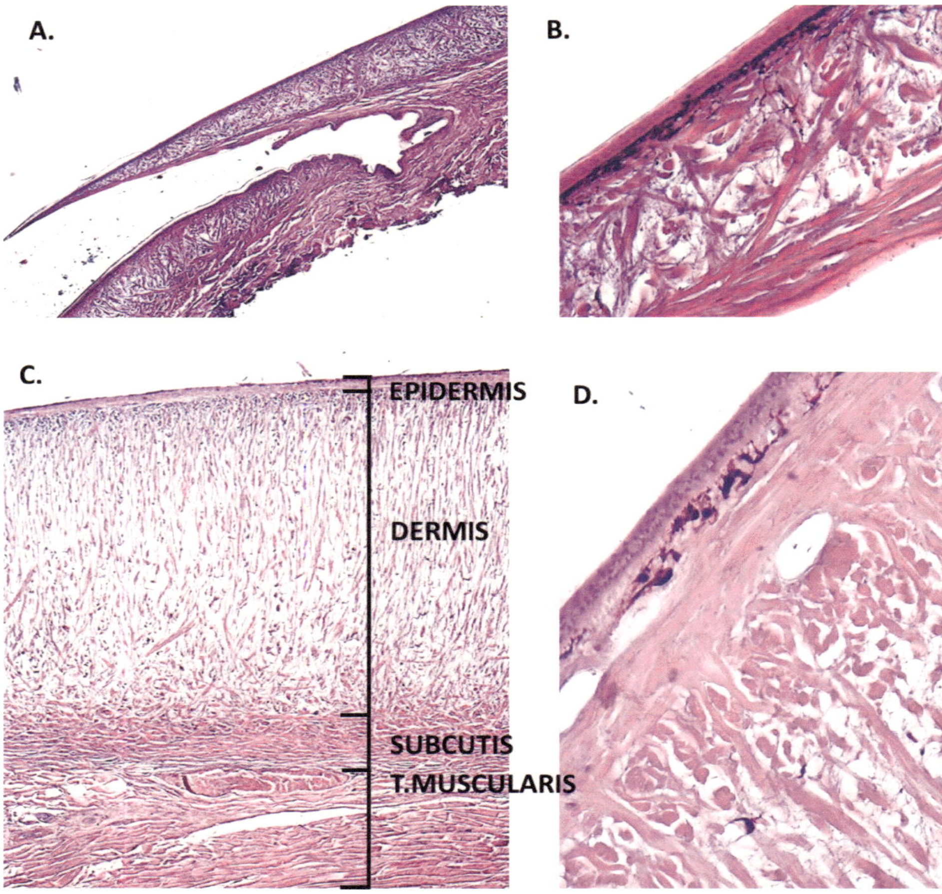

Figure 10.
Skin histology of the tail (A, B) and ventral part (B, D) of Burmese Python (Python bivittatus). Skin from the tail and ventral part of the Burmese Python was stained with H&E staining. The sample was taken in the resting stage of the epidermis, when the animal was not in the process of ecdysis. In epidermis, the most visible part is the basal layer with keratinocytes with nuclei, which are dividing with mitosis. In figure (A) and (B), the existence of the overlapping scales and hinge region is observed. The melanin pigment is not evenly spread on all surfaces of scales. Mostly, it is observed in the overlapping scale and much less from the hinge region to the scale, which is overlapped. Approximately five layers were identified by microscopic observation. These were the oberhautchen, β-layer, the mesos layer, α-layer, and dermis. The β- and α-layers consisted of cells which become keratinized with the production of two types of keratin (β- and α-keratins). The oberhautchen did not show smooth characteristics, followed the inner scale surface and hinge region composed of thin β-layer. At the abdominal part of the skin, the epidermis is thicker. Dermis contains many more melanophores. In the dermis, fibrous connective tissue, vessels, nerves, melanophores, and Merkel mechanoreceptor cells are observed. In dermis connective tissue together with collagen fibers hard interesting pattern, which was distinctive in both samples. (A) 100× magnification, (B) 400× magnification.

develop inside the last one and before the skin is shed, the tip of new button shrinks. This process continues, and an appendage consists of a number of interlocking segments that sound characteristically. The sound is generated by friction one button to another, especially when snake feels endangered. In grass snakes (*Natrix natrix*), pine snakes (*Pituophis spp.*), and kingsnakes (*Lampropeltis spp.*), similar sounds are produced as heard in rattlesnakes by shaking their tail or other body parts against the surface where they are [27].

Snakes periodically molt their scaly skins and acquire new ones. This permits replacement of old worn out skin, disposal of parasites, and is thought to allow the snake to grow. The shape and arrangement of scales are used to identify snake species [14].

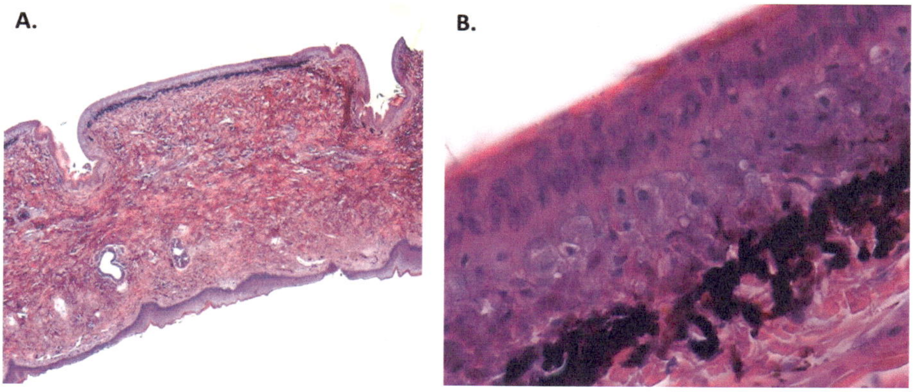

Figure 11.
Skin histology of the lip of the Emerald Tree Boa (Corallus caninus). Skin from the lip of the Emerald Tree Boa was stained with H&E staining. The sample was taken in the resting stage of the epidermis, when the animal was not in the process of ecdysis. In epidermis (B), the most visible part is the basal layer with keratinocytes containing nuclei, which are dividing under mitosis. Very visible is also the melanophore layer. This side is oriented toward the lip side. Keratinized epithelium (at the bottom of panel (A)) is more heavily keratinized and fewer melanophores are observed. (A, C) 100× magnification, (C, D) 400× magnification.

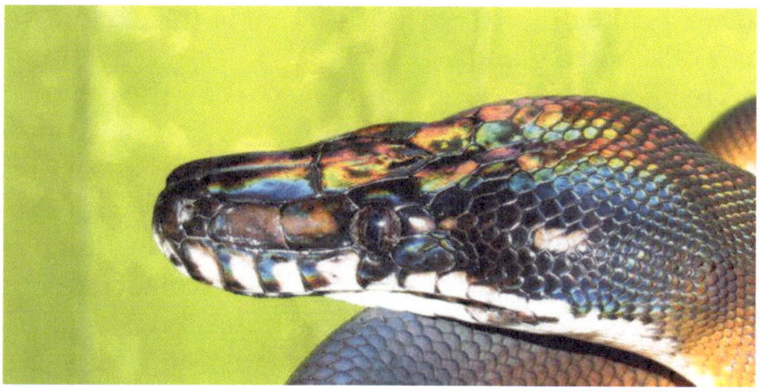

Figure 12.
Iridescence in white-lipped python (Liasis albertisii) (Photography Valentina Kubale).

5. Skin and scute features in crocodiles

In crocodiles and turtles, the dermal armor is formed from the deeper dermis rather than the epidermis and does not form the same sort of overlapping structure as snake scales. These dermal scales are more properly called scutes. Similar dermal scutes are found in the feet of birds and tails of some mammals and are believed to be the primitive form of dermal armor in reptiles [8].

The crocodile skin has horny plates, named scutes, in which shape, number, and position are important for the identification of the species. They can also become similar to bones and form an outer bone armor. The horny plates on the back are referred as the back shield, and below are dermal plates (4–10 longitudinal plates whose number varies depending on the animal species). On the abdominal side beneath the horny scutes, there are no bone plates. On the tail, scutes form rings with two rows continuing in one row of scutes by the end of the tail. The position of the horny scutes on the head is characteristic for each animal species. On the head beneath the horny scutes, bone plates are located. Unlike other reptiles, crocodiles do not shed their scutes, and they are renewed by scrubbing against different outer surfaces [28].

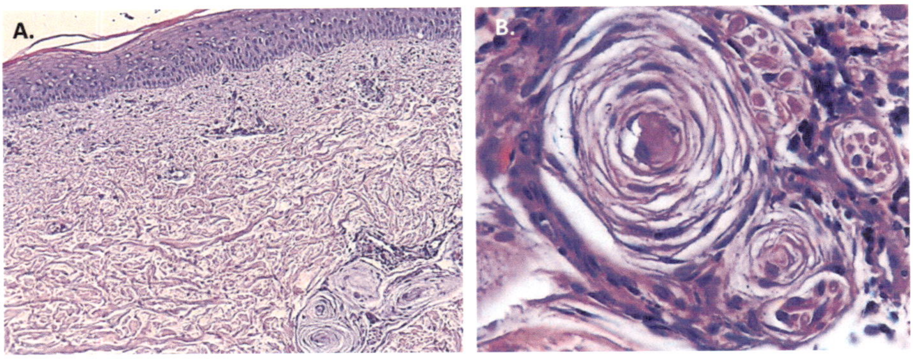

Figure 13.
Skin histology of the lip of Cuvier's Dwarf Caiman (Paleosuchus palpebrosus), stained with H&E. (A) The epidermis and dermis are observed. Thick stratified epidermis consists of several layers with recognizable stratum basale and a few more layers with enucleated keratinocytes. Stratum corneum is thinner and more compact, especially above the ISO region. ISOs are in the dermis, between thick fibers of connective tissue, vessels, and nerves. Melanophores are not observed. Around ISO, multiple vessels and nerves are observed (B). ISO bodies are concentrically shaped, similar to mammals. (A) 100× magnification, (B) 400× magnification.

In the skin of the crocodile, pigmented cells are located that give a color that varies from green to light brown to gray. In most animals, the belly is lighter than the rest of the body. Scent glands in crocodiles open in the cloaca. Alligators of both sexes have one pair of scented glands.

Crocodiles can recognize the prey on land even when they are under water because their eyes are located dorsally on their heads. They have very well-developed hearing and vision. Their upper eyelids are more mobile than the bottom ones and there is a tarsal bone plate located in the lower eyelid, which can develop into bony structure in some years. The upper eyelids are used to close the eye. The crocodile has also developed a third eyelid containing a cartilage, covering the eye when the animal is under water. They have an external hole on the head that looks like a rasp to collect sounds from the environment and is closed with a fibrous moveable lid that closes the aperture when the animal dives [14].

A very interesting feature in the crocodilian skin is the higher density of "integumentary sensory organs" (ISOs) in their dermis, which are particularly dense in the mouth area and the facial part of the head. They contain multiple mechanoreceptors, which are innervated by the vast network of the peripheral nerves [29]. They are important for the detection of surface waves generated by the moving prey and important for regulating jaws closing, depending on the size of the prey [29, 30]. ISOs are observed as a common feature in the skin, observed as a lamellar body (**Figure 13**).

6. Turtles and their special skin features

In the turtle, there are free parts of the body, such as the head, legs, and tail, covered with scales. In a turtle, the skin's appearance varies from smooth skin, where we can hardly see scales, to thick and crusty skin, which depends on the adaptation and the way of life. Toward the neck, the skin is wrinkled. Because of the adaptation of the land-based lifestyle in the Testudinidae family, the thicker skin is visible, and the scales are more pronounced. Changing the scales in turtles is periodic and individual and is more pronounced in aquatic turtles [14].

The turtle skin consists of the superficial part (*epidermis*) and the inner layer (*dermis*). Between these two layers, there is a basal lamina (BL). The surface layer consists of three layers: *stratum basale*, *stratum granulosum*, and *stratum corneum*. In the *stratum basale,* new cells proliferate and replace old and dead cells and push them toward the surface of the skin. Epithelial cells, keratinocytes, which are found in the *stratum corneum*, produce the protein keratin, which plays a key role in reducing loss of water. On the parts of the body that are more exposed to mechanical pressure, the keratinized layer may be even thicker. There are no blood vessels in the skin epidermis, so the epidermis cells are fed by diffusion from the deeper layers of the skin through the BL. Apart from keratinocytes in the epidermis, melanocytes and Langerhans cells are also located there. Epidermis is developed from ectoderm, creates the BL, and has the function of retaining water in the body, as well as the protection against infections and harmful external influences. New cells created in *stratum basale* replace old and dead cells and suppress them at the surface of the skin. The skin dermis is derived from mesoderm and creates a reticular lamina (*lamina reticularis*). In this layer, there are many sensory nerves (nerve endings and mechanoreceptors) as well as glands, blood vessels, and lymph vessels. Subcutis is a fatty and slightly connective tissue (**Figure 14**).

In the turtle skin, horny plates are formed together with osteoderms. Dermal bones are found below in the inner part of the skin (*dermis*) and they grow together to gain more strength. Corneal scales are made of water-insoluble keratin, which are laid in the arrangement allowing a thin layer of skin between them that makes it easier for the animal to move. In tortoises, the osteoderms are grown together with the spine and ribs, thus forming the back of the armor, carapace. The back and abdomen of the armor, depending on the type of the turtle, consists of several bones (shields). Above the bones (osteoderms), there is a layer of skin (epidermis) which is in the turtles with soft shell (the genus Apalone, the genus of the turtle *Dermochelys*) "skinned." In the other turtles, above the bony plates, there are also horny plates, which do not entirely match the shells' strength and ability to regenerate [31].

Carapace is constructed from at least 38 corneal scutes, depending on the species of the turtle. In the middle of the carapace, along the back, there are vertebral or neural corneal scutes (mostly five). On the left and the right sides, the neural scutes have either bony or costal plates, and, laterally, there are marginal scutes. A series of smaller plates, which on the border with carapace and plastron,

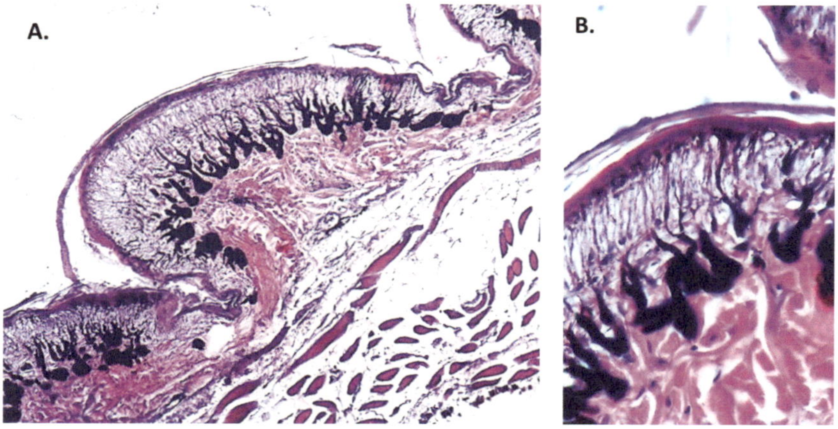

Figure 14.
Skin histology of the leg skin of the Red-ear slider (Trachemys scripta elegans), stained with H&E. On Panel A, epidermis and dermis are observed. Epidermis is thick and keratinized. It consists of several layers with recognizable stratum basale and a few more layers with enucleated keratinocytes. Stratum corneum is thick. In the dermis, vast melanophores are observed along with a thick layer of dense connective tissue, together with blood vessels and nerves. Subcutis consists of gentile connective tissue, and, in the tunica muscularis, skeletal muscles cells are observed (A) 100× magnification, (B) 400× magnification.

are called inframarginal scutes. Cranial from the first neural scutes it is nuchal plate. Above the tail are two scutes named suprapygeal (supracaudal). In the intramarginal plates, Rathke's pores are visible in sea turtles and similar structures can be observed in freshwater turtles. Below Rathke's pores, Rathe's glands are located, covered with fat tissue [31, 32]. The plastron is the nearly flat part of the shell structure of a turtle, which is basically the ventral surface of the shell. It also includes within its structure the anterior and posterior bridge struts and the bridge of the shell [32]. The plastron is made up of nine bones and the two epiplastra. The plastron usually consists of 12 plastral scutes, six on each side, which come together in the central line and their number depends on the shape of the shell and the type of turtle. Plastral formula is consisted from intergular, gular, humeral, pectoral, abdominal, femoral, and anal plastral scutes. The shape and mutual relationship of these scutes are of great importance in determining the species. In addition to the armor, turtles may also have specifically deployed jaw shells that may also be important in identifying the species. For example, in the sea turtles between the eyes, there are two horned shells that are characteristic of the Green sea turtle (*Chelonia mydas*), while in the other species there are more or only one. In the turtle, the dormant scutes are shed individually [14, 32].

In some turtles, fragrant glands are open in the cloaca, and in some species, they produce an intensive smell, especially when they feel endangered. For most skin glands, it is considered to play a major role in reproduction or defense against predators. In the terrestrial turtles, glands are located only on the thighs, while in the water turtles, the mucous glands are found along the skin. During the hibernation of turtles, gas exchange occurs through the skin, while being buried in the ground or for example at the bottom of the lake. The turtles have developed lacrimal glands (*gll. lacrimalis*) and Harder's glands that, like lacrimal glands, produce tears and contain immunocompetent cells. In the sea turtles, the lacrimal gland has been altered and modified into the solitary gland. The turtles do not have nasolacrimal ducts (*ductus nasolacrimalis*) and tears are secreted by evaporation.

7. Ecdysis

The shedding of scales is called *ecdysis*, trivially mostly named molting or sloughing. Sloughing serves number of functions. Firstly, the old and worn skin is replaced and secondly it helps to get rid of parasites (mites and ticks). In the epidermis, which is generally consisted of *stratum basale*, *stratum granulosum*, and *stratum corneum*, during the process prior to molting in the reptiles that slough large pieces of cornified skin layer changes occur [8].

In snakes, the complete outer layer of skin is shed in one piece and layer. During molting, most animals also change their behavior, they prefer to hide or move to a safe place and refuse food. In snakes, a thin skin layer in the form of a thin transparent membrane (*spectaculum*) covers their eyes; therefore, before sloughing, their vision is the weakest, as they have cloudy eyes which become bluish in color. This affects their behavior, and because of their faint vision, they become more nervous. The snakes become restless and begin to rub on uneven surfaces [1]. Just before shedding, the color of the skin becomes dull, colorless, and dry looking and the eyes become cloudy or blue-colored. Skin sloughing depends on many factors, such as growth rate, season, hibernation, mating, etc. Molting is repeated periodically throughout a snake's life. Wild animals slough two to four times a year (younger, still growing snakes may shed up to four times a year and later only twice), which in captivity can occur more often. The most common complications in captivity occur due to reduced humidity in the vivarium. The skin has no role in changing the gases except in the marine snakes that alternate the gases through the skin. When sloughing, they help themselves by rubbing at different surfaces. The old skin breaks near the mouth and the snake wriggles out, aided by rubbing against rough surfaces. In many cases, the cast skin peels backward over the body from head to tail, in one piece like an old sock. A new, larger, and brighter layer of skin forms underneath [14].

Snake scales are not discrete but are extensions of the epidermis; hence, they are not shed separately but are ejected as a complete contiguous outer layer of skin during each molt, similar to a sock being turned inside out. During the sloughing of the snake, the *stratum basale* is creating new cells, doubling *stratum granulosum* and *stratum corneum*. Specific to snakes and other reptiles is the formation of a *stratum intermedium*, a temporary layer between old and new skin. In this part of the skin, white blood cells help to separate layers and getting rid of the old layer of skin. Due to the pushing of old skin, the *stratum basale* is duplicated and after sloughing, the skin is up to 20% larger. Before the snakes shed the old skin, a new layer is already formed underneath it. The process of changing skin, takes about 2 weeks. As snakes grow, their skin cannot keep up with their growth, so they occasionally shed the skin (**Figure 15**).

In the case of lizards, this coating is shed periodically, usually coming off in flakes, but in some cases, such as lizards having elongated bodies, in a single piece. Some geckos will eat their own shed skin. Ecdysis is controlled by the thyroid gland. Changes in feeding behavior and activity occur prior to ecdysis and the reptiles become very susceptible to dehydration. Snakes tend to shed the whole skin, unlike lizards and chelonians which shed pieces, which makes them more vulnerable during ecdysis. In a healthy snake, the whole process can take up to about

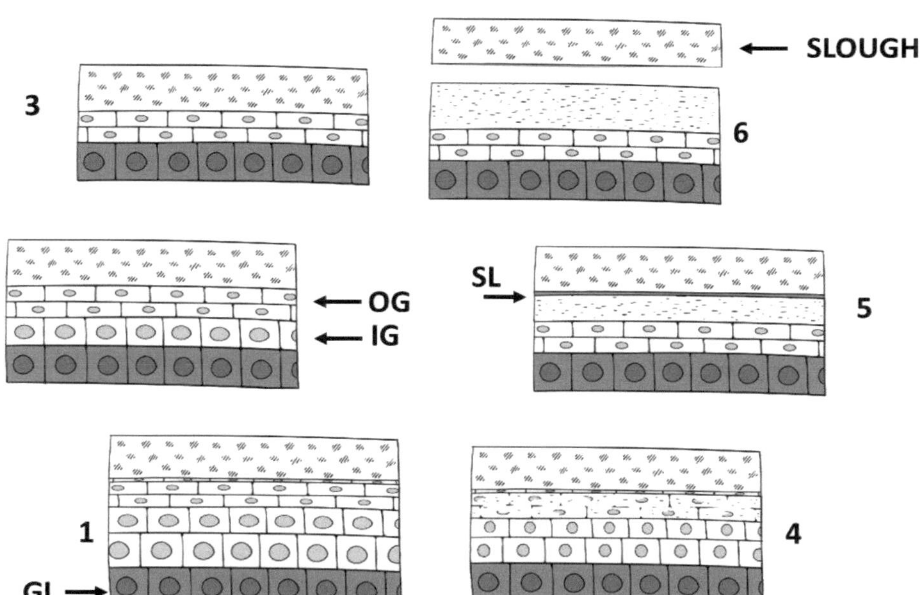

Figure 15.
Mechanism of the ecdysis in snakes (adopted from Kardong [8], designed by Pia Cigler). In lizards and snakes, the shedding of the cornified layer is called molting or ecdysis and results in the removal of the superficial epidermis. As molting begins, stratum basale, which has given rise to the strata granulosum (inner) and corneum (outer), duplicates the deeper layers of granulosum and corneum, pushing up under the old layers. During ecdysis, the cells in the intermediate layer replicate to form a new three-layer epidermis. Once this process is complete, lymph and white blood cells diffuse into the area between the two layers, and enzymes are released to form cleavage zone at the separation line. At this phase, the snake becomes gray, and snakes and lizards without the eyelids are also blind, because cornea is also changed. The old skin is shed, and the new epithelium hardens, decreasing permeability to become a new skin. GL—germinative layer, IG—inner generation of epidermis, OG—outer generation of epidermis, SL—separation line, S—slough.

2 weeks [8, 32]. In turtles and crocodiles, sloughing of the skin arises to a lesser extent and it is comparable to that of birds and mammals, in whom small flakes fall off at irregular intervals and it takes longer periods.

8. Clinical importance of histology and anatomy knowledge for the dermatology of reptiles

Reptile skin heals much slower than mammalian skin, often taking about 6 weeks to fully restore the defect. Malnourished animals are hypoproteinemic and unable to produce enough enzymes to form true cleavage zone, resulting in dysecdysis (failure to shed). Lack of moisture will also delay the process [11]. Skin permeability increases when skin is in contact with water, so water baths are a good way to rehabilitate sick reptiles and treat dysecdysis [11]. Wound healing is slow in reptiles, so stitches should be left at least 6 weeks [32]. It is best to leave stitches in place until ecdysis occurs since the increased activity in the dermis in epidermis promotes better healing and strength.

It should also be considered that during ecdysis, the skin becomes more permeable and more vulnerable to parasites and infection.

9. Materials and methods for histology sections

Samples of the skin tissue of different reptile species were preserved in 5% formaldehyde. Pieces of different types of tissue were included in the paraffin by using usual procedure with the apparatus Leica TP1020. Histological slides were prepared before use by the procedure which ensured that histological sections adhered to the slides properly and prevented sections from falling off the slides during further procedures. Tissue samples embedded in paraffin were cut by a hand microtome (Leica) into 5-μm-thick slices, which were transferred with brushes onto the smooth surface of warm water bath (40°C) and from there on the microscopic slides. Histological slides were dried in a thermostat (50°C). For classical histological staining with hematoxylin-eosin (H&E), samples were deparaffinized in xylene substitute (Neoclear; Merck) (2 × 5 minutes) and afterward rehydrated in decreasing concentrations of ethyl alcohol (100% for 2 × 5 minutes, 96% for 5 minutes, 75% for 5 minutes) and distilled water (2 × 5 minutes). In the following steps, samples were stained with either hematoxylin (Merck) (2 minutes), washed in running water (20 minutes), stained with eosin (1–2 minutes), and washed in distilled water (5 minutes) or Toluidine blue dye solution (20 minutes) and washed in distilled water (5 minutes) three times. Further, dehydration in ethyl alcohol with increasing concentration was performed (75% for approximately 5 minutes [depending on the sample; appropriate timing is observed during staining for intensity of reaction], 96% for 1× around 5 minutes, 100% for 2 × 5 minutes). Clarification of samples after drying and staining was carried out in xylene substitute (Neoclear) (3 × 5 minutes). At the end, a drop of Neo-Mount medium (Merck) was applied onto each tissue sample and the sample was covered with cover slide. Pictures were taken on Nikon FXA microscope with Nikon DS-F1 camera and transferred to program for image analysis by Lucia-G.

Acknowledgements

Authors would like to acknowledge financial support from ARRS, Research group P4-0053; Jasna Šporar for technical assistance with histological samples;

Prof. Alenka Dovč and Zlatko Golob, PhD, for their help with providing diverse reptile samples; and Catrin S. Rutland for winning the Women in Science award, which resulted in us preparing this chapter and book, and for English language proof-reading.

Author details

Catrin Sian Rutland[1], Pia Cigler[2] and Valentina Kubale[3*]

1 School of Veterinary Medicine and Science, University of Nottingham, Leicestershire, UK

2 Small Animal Clinic, Service for Birds and Reptiles, University of Veterinary Medicine Vienna, Austria

3 Veterinary Faculty, Institute for Preclinical Sciences, University of Ljubljana, Ljubljana, Slovenia

*Address all correspondence to: valentina.kubale@vf.uni-lj.si

References

[1] Chang C, Wu P, Baker RE, Maini PK, Alibardi L, Chuong CM. Reptile scale paradigm: Evo-Devo, pattern formation and regeneration. The International Journal of Developmental Biology. 2009;**53**(5-6):813-826

[2] Coborn J. The Atlas of Snakes of the World. New Jersey: TFH Publications; 1991

[3] Bauer AM, Kluge AG, Schuett G. Lizards. In: Halliday A, Adler K, editors. The Firefly Encyclopedia of Reptiles and Amphibians. Ontario: Firefly Books; 2002. pp. 139-169

[4] Starr C, Taggart R, Evers C. Biology: The Unity and Diversity of Life. Boston: Cengage Learning; 2012. p. 429

[5] Hickman C, Roberts L, Keen S, Larson A, l'Anson H, Eisenhour D. Integrated Principles of Zoology. 14th ed. Boston, MA: McGraw-Hill; 2006. 910 p

[6] Hickman C, Roberts L, Keen S. Animal Diversity. 6th ed. New York: McGraw Hill; 2012. 479 p

[7] Alibardi L. Aaptation to the land: The skin of reptiles in comparison to that of amphibians and endotherm amniotes. Journal of Experimental Zoology Part B: Molecular and Developmental Evolution. 2003;**298**(1):12-41

[8] Kardong KV. Vertebrates, Comparative Anatomy, Function, Evolution. 3rd ed. New York: McGraw-Hill; 2002

[9] Bellairs A The Life of Reptiles, The Skin. Vol. 2. London: Weidenfeld and Nicolson; 1969. pp. 283-332

[10] Lillywhite HB, Maderson PF. Skin structure and permeability. In: Gans C, Pugh FH, editors. Biology of the Reptilia, Physiology C. Vol. 12. London: Academic Press; 1982. pp. 397-433

[11] Price ER. The physiology of lipid raft storage and use in reptiles. Biological Reviews. 2017;**92**:1406-1426

[12] Bauer AM, Russel AP, Shadwick RE. Mechanical properties and morphological correlates of fragile skin in gekkonid lizards. The Journal of Experimental Biology. 1989;**145**:79-102

[13] Kubale V, editor. Skrb za zdravje eksotičnih živali v sožitju s človekom: informativni priročnik za lastnike živali in študijsko gradivo za študente veterinarstva, izd. Vol. 1. Ljubljana: Veterinarska fakulteta; 2018. 212 p

[14] Gravish N, Autumn K. Gecko adhesion: Evolutionary nanotechnology. Philosophical Transactions of the Royal Society A. 2008;**366**:1575-1590

[15] Hamasaki DI. Properties of the parietal eye of the green iguana. Vision Research. 1968;**8**(5):591-599

[16] Teyssier J, Saenko SV, van der Marel D, Milinkovitch MC. Photonic crystals cause active colour change in chameleons. Nature Communications. 2015;**6368**(6):1-7

[17] Duarte RC, Flores AVF, Stevens M. Camouflage through colour change: Mechanisms, adaptive value and ecological significance. Philosophical Transactions of the Royal Society of London. Series B, Biological Sciences. 2017;**372**(1724):20160342

[18] Stuart-Fox D, Moussalli A. Selection for social signalling drives the evolution of chameleon colour change. PLoS Biology. 2008;**6**(1):e25

[19] Ligon RA, McGraw KJ. Chameleons communicate with complex colour changes during contests: Different body regions convey different information. Biology Letters. 2013;**9**:20130892

[20] Dost U. Chamäleons. 2 Auflage ed. Stuttgart: Ulmer Eugen; 2007

[21] Krey K, Farayalah A. Skin histology and microtopography of Papuan White Snake (*Micropechis ikaheka*) in relation to their zoogeographical distribution. HAYATI Journal of Biosciences. 2013;**20**(1):7-19

[22] Hazel J, Stone M, Grace S, Tsukruk VT. Nanoscale design of snake skin for reptation locomotions via friction anisotropy. Journal of Biomechanics. 1999;**32**(5):477-484

[23] Toni M, Alibardi L. Soft epidermis of a scaleless snake lacks beta-keratin. European Journal of Histochemistry. 2007;**51**:145-151

[24] Klein MC, Gorb SN. Epidermis architecture and material properties of the skin of four snake species. Journal of the Royal Society Interface. 2012;**9**:3140-3155

[25] Reiserer RS, Schuet WG. Chapter 7: The origin and evolution of the rattlesnake rattle: Misdirection, clarification, theory, and progress. In: Schuett GW, Feldner MJ, Smith CF, Reiserer RS, editors. Rattlesnakes of Arizona. Vol. 2. Rodeo, New Mexico: ECO Publishing; 2016. pp. 245-276

[26] Stidworthy J. Snakes of the World. New York: Grosset & Dunlap Inc.; 1969. 160 p

[27] Chen IH, Yang W, Meyers MA. Alligator osteoderms: Mechanical behavior and hierarchical structure. Materials Science & Engineering. C, Materials for Biological Applications. 2014;**35**:441-448

[28] Leitch DB, Catania KC. Structure, innervation and response properties of integumentary sensory organs in crocodilians. Journal of Experimental Biology. 2012;**215**:4217-4230

[29] Di-poi N, Milinkovitch MC. Crocodilians evolved scattered multi-sensory micro-organs. Evolutionary Developmental Biology. 2013;**4**:19

[30] Zangerl R. The turtle shell. In: Gans C, Bellairs DA, Parsons TA, editors. Biology of the Reptilia, Morphology A. Vol. 1. London: Academic Press; 1969. pp. 311-340

[31] Cordero GA. The turtle's shell. Current Biology. 2017;**27**(5):R168-R169

[32] O'Malley B. Clinical Anatomy and Physiology of Exotic Species. Structure and Function of Mammals, Birds, Reptiles and Amphibians. Philadelphia: Saunders Ltd.; 2005